Spirituality and Coping with Loss

End of Life Healthcare Practice

Spirituality and Coping with Loss

End of Life Healthcare Practice

Wendy Greenstreet

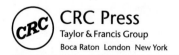

CRC Press
Taylor & Francis Group
Boca Raton London New York

CRC Press is an imprint of the
Taylor & Francis Group, an **informa** business

CRC Press
Taylor & Francis Group
6000 Broken Sound Parkway NW, Suite 300
Boca Raton, FL 33487-2742

© 2016 by Taylor & Francis Group, LLC
CRC Press is an imprint of Taylor & Francis Group, an Informa business

No claim to original U.S. Government works

Printed on acid-free paper
Version Date: 20151211

International Standard Book Number-13: 978-1-78523-148-3 (Paperback)

Library of Congress Cataloging-in-Publication Data

Names: Greenstreet, Wendy, author.
Title: Spirituality and coping with loss : end of life healthcare practice / Wendy Greenstreet.
Description: Boca Raton : Taylor & Francis, 2016. | Includes bibliographical references and index.
Identifiers: LCCN 2015048580| ISBN 9781785231483 (paperback : alk. paper) | ISBN 9781498767835 (e-book) | ISBN 9781498767842 (e-book-vital book) | ISBN 9781498767859 (epub)
Subjects: | MESH: Spiritual Therapies--nursing | Terminal Care--methods | Spirituality | Bereavement | Nurse's Role
Classification: LCC RZ401 | NLM WY 152.3 | DDC 615.8/52--dc23
LC record available at http://lccn.loc.gov/2015048580

**Visit the Taylor & Francis Web site at
http://www.taylorandfrancis.com**

**and the CRC Press Web site at
http://www.crcpress.com**

Printed and bound by CPI Group (UK) Ltd, Croydon, CR0 4YY

Contents

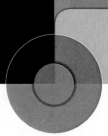

Acknowledgements

I would like to express my thanks to the nurses who gave their time to participate in this research, and their managers who facilitated access and provided space for interviews to take place. I have appreciated many forms of support resourced by Canterbury Christ Church University. Special gratitude and sincere thanks are warranted for the late Professor Sue Holmes, whose encouragement accounts for my undertaking this research, and whose support was generous in its availability, and much valued on my part. Thanks also to Dr Tim Clark, who has patiently guided me through the challenges of phenomenological methodology. I would also like to express my appreciation to Dr Doug MacInness for his support in Sue's absence. Importantly, I must thank my husband Graham for his stalwartness throughout this endeavour, and my son and daughter, Ben and Sophie, for their encouragement.

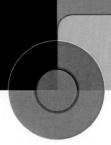

About the author

Dr Wendy Greenstreet commenced this research while a Principal Lecturer in Nursing at Canterbury Christ Church University. She qualified as an RGN in 1978 and as an RNT in 1983. Research to complete an MA(Ed) triggered an enduring interest in teaching spirituality in nursing and later in health and social care. A second specialist interest in issues of loss lead to further postgraduate study in psychosocial palliative care, followed by the development and delivery of post-registration and postgraduate curriculum in palliative care. Wendy has moved her dual interest in spiritual care and loss forward in this PhD study. She remains an associate of Canterbury Christ Church University.

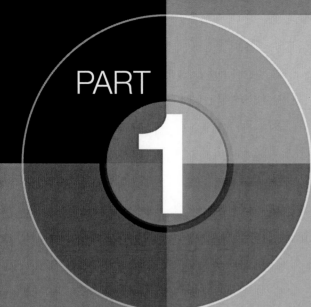

PART 1

SETTING THE SCENE

My interest in spirituality as a concept relevant initially to nursing practice and more recently health and social care, was triggered by practical need. The 1980s had seen changes in the nursing curriculum, embracing a more holistic focus on care, and had incorporated the social and psychological needs of patients alongside the very well-established focus on physical care. However, it was not until 1990 that the curriculum included patients' spiritual needs as a constituent of holistic care. An evaluative study of the effectiveness of my teaching spirituality in the pre-registration programme followed. This provided evidence that progression in achieving learning after theoretical input on spirituality was largely sustained on evaluation 18 months later. I went on to find post-registration students, studying the human experience of disability, avidly interested in spirituality as a concept concerned with meaning and making sense of situations. They readily related to issues concerning ultimate questions in which patients wanted to know 'why' disability had happened to them.

Later, I undertook postgraduate study of psychosocial palliative care, which was followed by my development of curriculum that included modules on loss in post-registration and postgraduate programmes. Significant loss challenges our assumptive world and potentially creates a spiritual crisis,[1] in generating a search to make sense of unwanted change that has been thrust upon us. The questions asked by those living with chronic and terminal illness have a similar ring to the questions explored by those post-registration nurses considering spirituality and the human experience of disability. Collectively these experiences have brought me to this research, to gain a better understanding of spirituality in relation to coping with loss in situations of advanced chronic or terminal illness.

REFERENCE

1. Agrimson LB and Taft LB. Spiritual crisis, a concept analysis. *Journal of Advanced Nursing.* 2008; **65**(2): 454–61.

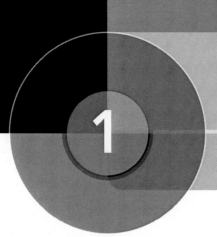

Introduction: the point of the study

1

This book gives an account of a study situated in the South East of England, and explores practising nurses' experience of spirituality as a resource in end of life care. Coping in end of life care situations often involves both a sense of loss as well as actual loss. Although my experiences as an educationalist brought me to this research, the justification for the study was grounded on more than practice experience and personal interest; it was also congruent with government policy on healthcare development.

Hospice care is accessible to a minority of patients and almost exclusively to those with cancer. The Department of Health working paper on end of life care strategy[1] reflected an increasing emphasis on the need for the principles of care exemplified in hospice to be made available to those with advanced chronic and terminal illness in all settings. The working paper acknowledged that many patients had unmet spiritual and psychological needs, and that their carers had similar needs, both during the patient's illness and in bereavement. It also predicted that the emergent End of Life Care Strategy would need to focus not only on 'what' should be done but also 'how'. The End of Life Care Strategy[2] that followed ratified these proposals in aiming to bring high-quality care to all people approaching the end of life, and proposing that this should be available both at home and in institution settings. Further affirmation was evident in the strategy's 10 objectives, one of which specified that all those approaching the end of life have access to physical, psychological, social and spiritual care.

AIM AND OBJECTIVES

The aim of the study was to explore nurses' lived experience of spirituality as a means of helping patients to cope with loss associated with terminal or chronic disease. The study objectives were threefold. First, to gain an understanding of nurses' perceptions of spirituality as an aspect of person-centred care, second, to explore the extent to which nurses facilitate spirituality as a source of coping, and finally, to explore how nurses use their personal resources in caring for those with chronic and terminal conditions. Research participants were recruited from community, care home and hospice settings where these patients are cared for.

Central to the concept of spirituality in healthcare is a concern with, and an attempt to make sense of, circumstances and outcomes of illness. In situations of loss, whether associated with chronic disease, degenerative disease or terminal illness and bereavement, individuals seek to know: why? Questions of meaning are likely to be complex. In linking past research on spirituality in healthcare with studies on loss and bereavement associated with professional roles, this study furthers knowledge of nurses' responses to spiritual questions and how they apply these to their professional practice.

RESEARCH DESIGN

A study that links spirituality and coping in healthcare contexts is suited to a qualitative research design in its attempt to discover nurses' experience, and thus generate an understanding of their roles in this aspect of care. Phenomenology is a qualitative methodology in which meanings are a key to the study of an individual's experience.[3] The association of the concept of spirituality with a search for meaning[4] sits well with the phenomenological stance that experience is one of interrelated meanings which collectively constitute the world as we know it, our 'lifeworld'.

The style of phenomenology used as methodology is determined by the stance the researcher takes in the study. Descriptive forms of phenomenology require the researcher to attempt to put aside all knowledge and experience they have of the phenomena that are the focus of their study in order to describe the experience of participants without being influenced by their own preconceptions. On the other hand, interpretative forms of phenomenology accept that the knowledge and experience of the phenomena which are the focus of study have influenced the researcher's choice of study and will influence their interpretation of participant experience. Spirituality is such an integral part of us, core to our very personhood,[5] that consequently any attempt to try to step outside of our experience of this phenomenon is unrealistic. Therefore, Chapter 2 addresses the particular form of interpretative phenomenology chosen as the approach best suited to this study.

Interpretative forms of phenomenology require that I explain my situation in relation to the research topic and its participants. In this way, I remain conscious of how my previous knowledge and experience influence my interpretation of data. For this reason, Chapter 3 presents a literature review that reflects the synthesis of my scholarship and experience prior to this research.

How and why research participants were identified through purposive sampling of nurses involved with end of life care in hospice, community and care home settings within South East England is explained in Chapter 4. Exclusion criteria included acute settings, practice contexts where patient throughput is rapid, and those outside of South East England. The size of the sample was determined by the number of participants interviewed until adequacy of data was reached. Interviews obtaining descriptions of participants' experience of spirituality in relation to coping with loss were the primary means of data collection. The use of a topic guide helped direct conversation toward the phenomena studied, and resulted in interviews being designated as semi-structured.

The stepped approach to analysis of data described in Chapter 5 closely reflects the scheme of Smith *et al.*[6] and provides a tool to address the process of engaging with, and interpreting the meaning of, the 'lived experience' documented in the transcripts of semi-structured interviews with the participants. This process starts by looking at one transcript and then moving on to the others one by one. The emergent themes are then listed to facilitate the analytical or theoretical ordering necessary to elicit connections between them. Some consideration of reflexivity and analysis of my diary documenting reflection on the research process is also included in this chapter.

FINDINGS AND IMPLICATIONS

Study findings are addressed in two sections. Part 2 comprises chapters that consider the impact of loss as a context of care. Part 3 contains those chapters which examine the impact of the process of care on nurses' proficiency in spiritual care. The implications of these findings for education and practice are addressed in the chapters that constitute Part 4.

SUMMARY

There are an increasing number of studies that consider spirituality in healthcare and how patients' spiritual needs can be recognized and fulfilled. However, this study provides a different perspective. In particular, it illuminates what and how nurses contribute to these aspects of care in situations of loss, in both institutional and community settings. It also considers how nurses, as professional carers, cope with their own existential questioning in the face of others' suffering

REFERENCES

1. Department of Health. *Working Paper End of Life Strategy.* London: Department of Health, 2006.
2. Department of Health. *End of Life Care Strategy: Promoting High Quality Care for All Adults at the End of Life.* London: Department of Health, 2008.
3. Ashworth P. The origins of qualitative psychology. In: Smith JA, editor. *Qualitative Psychology a Practical Guide to Research Methods.* London: Sage, 2003, 4–24.
4. Greenstreet W. Clarifying the concept. In: Greenstreet W, editor. *Integrating Spirituality in Health and Social Care: Perspectives and Practical Approaches.* Oxford: Radcliffe Publishing, 2006, 7–19.
5. Ibid.
6. Smith JA, Flowers P and Larkin M. *Interpretative Phenomenological Analysis, Theory, Method and Research.* London: Sage, 2009.

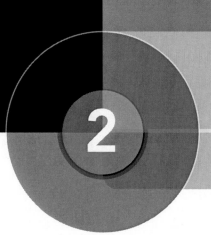

The choice of approach

The choice of approach to a study, its methodology, needs to reflect the nature of the research. In this case, a study focused on nurses' experience of spirituality as a resource in coping with loss was not one amenable to a positivist, or quantitative, approach. Positivist methodology would require quantification, or reduction of experiences of spirituality to a measurable form. Spirituality as a concept is abstract in nature, and so not only eludes literal description, but also evades quantifiable analysis.[1] Consequently, a qualitative research approach, emphasizing the quality of data rather than its quantity, quantification or measurability, was a more appropriate choice. This chapter explains the use of Heideggerian hermeneutics – and interpretative phenomenology influenced by Heideggerian philosophy – as my choice of qualitative methodology. The rationale for purposive sampling, use of semi-structured interviews as the method of data collection and the contribution of reflexivity to this study are also addressed.

PHENOMENOLOGY AS METHODOLOGY

Phenomenology seeks to understand another person's experience.[2] Experience is taken to reflect interrelated meanings that collectively constitute the world as we know it, our 'life-world'.[3] The style of phenomenology used as methodology is determined by the stance the researcher takes in the study. Descriptive forms of phenomenology are fundamentally based on the philosophy of Husserl[4] and require the researcher to attempt to put aside all knowledge and experience they have of the phenomena that are the subject of their study. This disciplined approach, known as 'bracketing', is considered necessary to ensure that the description of research participants' experience is not influenced by the researcher's preconceptions.[5] Alternatively, interpretative forms of phenomenology are fundamentally based on the philosophy of Heidegger[6] and accept that prior understanding on the part of the researcher[7] influences both the researcher's choice of phenomenon to study, and their interpretation of accounts of research participant experience.

I have explained how my scholarship and experience of promoting spirituality as a perspective of care in education settings have bought me to this research (see Part 1). Having immersed myself in subject matter related to both spirituality and loss for many years, it is unrealistic for me to contemplate 'bracketing', to set aside embedded knowledge. Instead, I am naturally drawn to the Heideggerian view of phenomenology, that my relevant experience has in fact seeded the study.

HEIDEGGERIAN HERMENEUTIC PHENOMENOLOGY

In our everyday experience life 'happens'; much of it comes about by chance, not all of it leaves an impression, but over time we acquire an accumulated knowledge and various skills that are meaningful – they have a recognizable function. Heidegger's philosophy sees phenomenology as the means of looking past the normal everyday meanings of life, to see the truth of our 'Being'.[8] 'Being' in this sense concerns our very essence and is evident in our human existence.[9] In 'Being' we are self-conscious, and so aware of our existence, and know our own fate as finite, and mortal.[10] Most research methodologies are epistemological in that they are concerned with the method, validity and scope of knowledge,[11] but as Heideggerian phenomenology is concerned with the study of our 'Being', it is described as ontological.

Central to Heidegger's philosophy is an interest in experience of phenomenon 'being-in-the-world'. Consequently, the meaning of experience of a phenomenon, for example spirituality as a resource in coping with loss, is seen to be related to context, the 'world' in which it occurs – in this case, situations of loss in end of life care environments. This is true for both the research participant and the researcher.[12] Hence my experience of addressing spirituality and loss with healthcare students in education forums is brought to research interviews with nurses who bring their experience of spirituality and loss from practice in end of life care environments. The intent of a Heideggerian methodological approach is therefore to interpret meaning already implicit in lived experience.[13] It is primarily a way of approaching research, rather than a specific, unique method. It involves using hermeneutics as the means of interpretation and understanding of all forms of communication, and thus includes written, oral, verbal and non-verbal communication.[14] In this way, transcripts of in-depth interviews in which research participants share their experience of spirituality as a resource in coping with loss provide written text for me as the researcher to enter into dialogue with – and to continually question and interpret – its meaning.

The process of interpretation in Heideggerian phenomenology is associated with the notion of the 'hermeneutic circle'.[15] The circle starts with the assumption that in order to understand we need to start with ideas. These ideas are expressed in terms that suggest we already have some understanding of what we are trying to understand. In this way understanding becomes a development of what we have understood. Therefore interpretation is 'developed understanding'. Although interpretation is grounded in something we grasp in advance, it clarifies understanding and enlarges the ideas that initiated the 'hermeneutic circle'. Therefore through this process my understanding that led to the idea of linking the concepts of spirituality and loss is clarified and developed.

Gadamer,[16] a German philosopher who shared Heidegger's interest in hermeneutics, describes the interpretative process symbolized by the hermeneutic circle as one where the whole of a text (e.g. an interview transcript) is understood in terms of its parts, and the parts in terms of the whole. The anticipation of meaning (of the whole text) becomes actual understanding when parts (of the text) shift expectation of meaning (of the whole text). This constant movement of understanding from whole to part, and back to whole text, reflects the shift in understanding that is interpretation.

Hermeneutic phenomenology acknowledges language as a tool central to human culture, in that it enables us to shape our understanding of experience and ultimately our reality.[17] The way language is used – through intonation, modulation, the tempo of talking, the very way we speak – conveys our state of mind.[18] A hermeneutic focus on the meaning of language values poetry and metaphor as a means of expressing experience by transcending the limits of language. Stanworth[19] illustrates the use of metaphor to express meaning; in her study, termi-nally ill patients use metaphor as a means of expressing experience related to spirituality. She explains:

We emerge from and return to silence, but the liminality both of human knowledge and human existence is not a 'puzzle' to be solved. It is a mystery with which we must live. Language only captures the surface of life (Ricouer 1976) and human existence carries degrees of meaning that exceed any interpretation – not as an 'add-on' but as a permeating dimension. The 'stranger' dwells in the heart of the familiar because, at life's deepest moments, something – which is no 'thing' – escapes articulation…to be concerned… with spirituality is not to be concerned with special events but akin to the artist, with the ordinary at a depth where conventional interpretations are relativized. Just as no painting is reducible to its brush strokes or any poem to the sum of its sentences…the artist's struggle to achieve…the moment of language going beyond itself…demonstrates a fidelity to the experiences of many patients, such as…Hazel pointing to her dying flowers as mediators of 'letting go' and personal dissolution, or Arthur's 'final salute', Debbie's 'inner flame', Tracy's statue and Mary's 'golden door' are not puzzles to be solved but ingenious resorts to the 'perspectival' character of poetic language…Metaphors are miniature acts of artistic creation or poiesis…(Rachel Stanworth. *Recognizing Spiritual Needs in People Who Are Dying.* 2004, 210–11. By permission of Oxford University Press.)

Benner[20] has used, and promoted, Heideggerian hermeneutics and interpretative phenom-enology influenced by Heideggerian philosophy as the methodology for nurse researchers studying nurses and nursing. Cohen and Omery[21] believe that current descriptions of her-meneutic approaches to research have abandoned Heidegger's philosophical quest for the meaning of 'Being', and so shifted away from ontological phenomenology. However, Benner's[22] view is that a hermeneutic, interpretative phenomenological research approach is ontological because the researcher is dealing with questions about why and how we know some things and not others, and what constitutes our knowing, rather than epistemological questions about what it is to know.

Benner[23] points out that the dialogical process needed to understand and interpret texts is an extension of the researcher's pre-existing abilities to understand the world and read texts for meaning. This ability is applied with rigour and attentiveness in interpretative research. She also points out that the need to engage reasoning in particular situations and particular texts is an approach that is seen to come more easily to nurses with some expertise, due to their practical knowledge about understanding and reading situations. Also, as nursing expertise evolves from experience that would include interviewing and eliciting a person's story in a wide range of settings, nurses are amenable to the role of storytelling as central to a hermeneutic approach to phenomenology. Storytelling allows people to structure and meaningfully give account for what they perceived as worth noting, their concerns and understanding of the situ-ation. Therefore nurse researchers' phenomenological interpretation of nurses' stories of lived experience potentially makes practical knowledge visible, and in so doing makes what Benner[24] describes as the knack, tact, craft and clinical knowledge inherent in expert nursing practice more accessible.

RATIONALE FOR METHOD

SAMPLE

Although sample size may be small in phenomenological research,[25] by purposively choosing participants whose experience is likely to involve or be impacted by issues of spirituality in situations of loss, data is more likely to provide in-depth information[26] and thus be rich and thick enough to facilitate adequate understanding of the phenomenon studied. Benner[27] is pragmatic in her approach to sample size in suggesting that it is limited by the size of the transcribed text produced in relation to the number of researcher hours available to analyse the text. She infers that sufficient text provides redundancy, clarity and confidence in the overall transcribed text, in that it will have covered an adequate range of situations. In addition, Benner[28] explains that sample size is adjusted depending on the quality of the text, and the way the lines of enquiry are shaped by participants. Criterion sampling works well when participants sought are those who have experience of the phenomenon.[29] Consequently, purposive sampling for this study involved choosing specific sites where staff who care for patients with chronic and terminal illness could be located and specifying a minimum requirement of post-registration practice experience for nurses to be eligible to participate.

INTERVIEWS

Phenomenological research focuses on the individual's own perspective, and assumes that reality is what participants perceive it to be.[30] For this reason interviews are often used to access participants' experience. Qualitative interviews use open questions.[31] In this way participants are able to use their own words to describe their experience. The purpose of interviews is to encourage dialogue to elicit participants' descriptions, perceptions, understandings and attribution of meaning to their experience.[32] The use of schedules or topic guides helps direct conversation toward the phenomena studied and results in interviews being designated as semi-structured. The art of listening to explicit descriptions and the meanings they convey needs to be complemented by what is said 'between the lines'. In reflecting their interpretation of what is said back to the participant in follow-up questions, the interviewer is often able to ascertain the accuracy of interpretation of data.[33]

Atkinson and Silverman[34] consider interviews are part of common culture, in that they provide a means of revealing the personal and private self, such as in television chat shows. However, they are potentially complex to administer because they involve skills of questioning, active listening, reflecting on answers and non-verbal cues, as well as the skilled use of verbal and non-verbal communication to sustain participant contribution to the focus of the research study.[35] Kvale and Brinkmann[36] suggest that qualitative research interviewing is a craft learnt through practice, which if done well can be considered an art. They consider a conversational style beneficial, and believe the quality of interviewing is evident in the strength and relevance of knowledge gathered. Interview knowledge is the product of the conversational relationship between interviewer and interviewee, each potentially learning from the other, or the active process of interview itself. This knowledge is described as actively created by questioning and response, and shaped or co-authored by interviewer and research participant. Consequently, qualitative interviewing often results in methodological decisions that need to be made as circumstances unfold during the interview itself.

Although relatively unstructured, there is asymmetry of power within qualitative interviews. This is partly because the interviewer determines the focus of topics explored, but also due to the 'professional' rather than 'everyday' nature of interview conversations.[37] Consequently it is important to consider the ethical implications of balancing the research interviewer's interest in probing for further in-depth knowledge, against the interviewee's interest in relation to self-disclosure.

REFLEXIVITY

Reflexivity relates to the researchers' awareness of the values and experiences that they bring to qualitative study.[38] It is often confused with reflection. Finlay[39] suggests that the terms are best considered as a continuum. She describes reflection as 'thinking about' something after the event, which is not dissimilar to Schon's[40] reflection-on-action or Johns'[41] reflection-on-experience involving a dialogue with self after the event. Finlay,[42] however, describes reflexivity as involving a more immediate, dynamic form of subjective self-awareness that continues throughout an event, such as an interview. This is more than Schon's[43] reflection-in-action, described by Johns as a form of impromptu problem solving 'on the hoof', but similar to Johns'[44] reflection-within-the-moment, where self-dialogue is conscious, but internalized as a response structured by reflective cues.

Finlay[45] acknowledges the value of reflexivity in enabling the researcher to recognize their interpretations, and ongoing revelation of the phenomenon studied. However, she also points out that it is the effectiveness of reflexive analysis that determines its value in research and warns against excessive reflexive introspection resulting in the researcher's voice overshadowing that of the participant.

RIGOUR

Interviews are subject to an interpersonal context, and therefore the nuances and meanings within the context of one interview may not be comparable with another.[46] Similarly, in relation to recordings of data gathered at interviews, there are many possible readings from each transcript.[47] Consequently, rather than refer to the traditional terms of reliability and validity associated with empirical studies, qualitative studies are concerned with issues of rigour in relation to dependability or truthfulness, which are evidenced in the presentation of an audit trail that clearly indicates the procedural steps of the study.[48]

Alaszewski[49] reviews published advice for guiding research participants completing diaries as part of empirical and naturalistic studies. Some of this advice is applicable to a diary kept by the researcher themselves 'alongside' their chosen method(s) of enquiry. Authenticity of account is critical, and unsolicited entries are an excellent resource in qualitative studies. The record of reflective thoughts and feelings concerning the study in a research diary contributes to making clear any issues of process. In this way, there is provision for transparency within the study to ensure that those who read it can decide if it is believable.[50]

ETHICAL CONSIDERATIONS

The ethical framework underpinning healthcare practice is rooted in deontology, which emphasizes professional duty.[51] However, there is a tension between this and a utilitarian view, which allows societal acknowledgement of autonomy in relation to the individual's right to decide. Kvale and Brinkmann[52] point out that these traditional ethical theories are reliant on principles and rules, which are not self-interpreting. Consequently, they do not determine when and how to apply the principles and rules they purport. Increasingly an alternative stance is proposed, that of virtue ethics, which are more concerned with the nature of the professional involved and their perception of the situation.[53] Therefore in the research interview situation rules and principles of traditional ethics are not so much abandoned but are considered as guides to help with reflection on ethical dilemma. Ethical responsibilities include academic integrity, honesty and respect for others.[54] Ethical consideration needs to be given to arrangements concerning access to participants, self-determination, autonomy and anonymity.

ANALYSIS

Hermeneutic analysis is by definition interpretative. Interpretative analysis is hinged on human activity being considered inherently meaningful. Schwandt[55] proposes three ways in which we can arrive at an understanding of the meaning of particular activity. The first of these is by empathetic identification, which involves trying to understand the research participant's motives, beliefs, desires and thoughts regarding the phenomena being explored. Gaining such an 'inside' understanding is acknowledged as central to the purpose of qualitative enquiry. The second is via phenomenological sociology, where interpretative analysis is concerned with understanding the everyday world that constitutes the participant's life. Conversation, interaction and reflexivity are the means of achieving this understanding. Third, language is a key to understanding significant systems of meanings, for example, cultural norms. With regard to this study, empathetic understanding of each participant's lived experience of spirituality – elicited in the interaction of conversation-style interviewing and reflexivity – is facilitated by my familiarity with the culture and language of nursing, the institutional norms and rules within healthcare, and my knowledge and understanding of spirituality.

Schwandt[56] goes on to describe philosophical hermeneutics as a fourth notion of analysis. This reflects, in principle, the process involved in the hermeneutic circle described earlier in this chapter. He proposes that understanding requires the engagement of our inherited bias and prejudice. In this way, bias and prejudice can be examined in the throes of interaction with participants, or in the analysis of texts of transcribed interviews, and altered to further our understanding of others as well as ourselves. Understanding is always bound up with language, in that preconceptions are tested in a dialogical encounter with what is not understood. Unlike other interpretative theorizing of understanding, which considers that human action has meaning that is determinable by the interpreter, in philosophical hermeneutics the text or human action is not an object that is simply discovered; instead, the interpretation of meaning is the understanding created by the interface of the perceiver's knowledge with the text or human action that constitutes research data.

SUMMARY

Phenomenology as methodology suits an enquiry that is interested in the research participants' experience, the 'world as they find it'. The choice of a Heideggerian hermeneutic phenomenological approach not only allows my familiarity with the phenomenon to be acknowledged but also allows that very familiarity to positively contribute to forming the research focus. Language is considered a tool which enables us to shape our understanding of experience. Participant stories of their experience of situations in which spirituality was a resource in coping with loss are shared at interview and captured in textual form as interview transcripts. In interpreting these texts, my reflexive awareness of the values and experience I bring to the study, together with my understanding of the language used, enable me to recognize my interpretations of data and elicit the meaning embodied in participants' 'lived experience'. In this way, I develop both enhanced and amended understandings of spirituality as a resource in coping with loss. Reflective thoughts recorded in my research diary provide a measure of the 'dependability' or 'truthfulness' of the study in accounting for issues of process.

REFERENCES

1. Stanworth R. *Recognising Spiritual Needs in People Who Are Dying.* Oxford: Oxford University Press, 2004.
2. Cohen MZ. Introduction. In: Cohen MZ, Kahn DL and Steeves RH, editors. *Hermeneutic Phenomenological Research: A Practical Guide for Nurse Researchers.* Thousand Oaks, London, New Delhi: Sage, 2000, 1–12.
3. Ashworth P. The origins of Qualitative Psychology. In: Smith JA, editor. *Qualitative Psychology: A Practical Guide to Research Methods.* London: Sage, 2003, 4–24.
4. Husserl E. *Ideas: General Introduction to Pure Phenomenology.* Translated by Boyce Gibson WR. London: George Allen and Unwin, 1931. (Originally published in German in 1913.)
5. Giorgi A and Giorgi B. Phenomenology. In: Smith JA, editor. *Qualitative Psychology: A Practical Guide to Research Methods.* London: Sage, 2003, 25–50.
6. Heidegger M. *Being and Time.* Translated by Macquarrie J and Robinson E. Oxford: Blackwell, 1962. (Originally published in German 1926.)
7. Polit DF and Beck CT. *Essentials of Nursing Research: Appraising Evidence for Nursing Practice.* London: Wolters Kluwer/Lippincott Williams & Wilkins, 2010.
8. Cohen MZ and Omery A. Schools of phenomenology: implications for research. In: Morse JM, editor. *Critical Issues in Qualitative Research Method.* London: Sage, 1994, 136–56.
9. Spiegelberg H. *The Phenomenological Movement: A Historical Introduction.* Volume 1. The Hague: Martinus Nijhoff, 1960.
10. Stokes P. *Philosophy, 100 Essential Thinkers.* London: Arcturus, 2005.
11. Pearsall J, editor. *The Concise Oxford Dictionary.* 10th ed. Oxford: Oxford University Press, 2001.
12. Cohen and Omery, op. cit.
13. Burch R. On phenomenology and its practices. *Phenomenology + Pedagogy.* 1989; **7**: 187–217.
14. Thiselton AC. Hermeneutics. In: Ferguson SB and Wright DF, editors. *New Dictionary of Theology.* Leicester: Inter-Varsity Press, 1988, 293–7.
15. Crotty M. *The Foundations of Social Research: Meaning and Perspective in the Research Process.* London: Sage, 1998.
16. Gadamer H-G. *Truth and Method.* 2nd revised ed. London: Sheed and Ward, 1989. Translated by Weinsheimer J and Marshall DG. (Originally published in German 1960.)
17. Crotty, op. cit.
18. Heidegger, op. cit.
19. Stanworth, op. cit.

20. Benner P. The tradition and skill of interpretative phenomenology in studying health, illness, and caring practices. In: Benner P, editor. *Interpretive Phenomenology: Embodiment, Caring, and Ethics in Health and Illness*. Thousand Oaks, CA: Sage, 1994, 99–127.
21. Cohen and Omery, op. cit.
22. Benner, op. cit.
23. Ibid.
24. Ibid.
25. Creswell JW. *Qualitative Inquiry and Research Design*. London: Sage, 2007.
26. Cohen, op. cit.
27. Benner, op. cit.
28. Ibid.
29. Creswell, op. cit.
30. Kvale S and Brinkmann S. *Interviews: Learning the Craft of Qualitative Research Interviewing*. Thousand Oaks, CA: Sage, 2009.
31. McLaughlin H. *Understanding Social Work Research*. London: Sage, 2007.
32. Jones SR and McEwen MK. A conceptual model of multiple dimensions of identity. In: Merriam SB *et al.*, editors. *Qualitative Research in Practice*. San Francisco, CA: Jossey-Bass, 2002, 163–74.
33. Kvale and Brickmann, op. cit.
34. Atkinson P and Silverman D. Kundera's immortality: the interview society and invention of self. *Qualitative Enquiry*. 1997; **3**: 304–25.
35. le May A, Holmes S. *Introduction to Nursing Research: Developing Research Awareness*. London: Hodder Arnold, 2012.
36. Kvale and Brickmann, op. cit.
37. Ibid.
38. Creswell, op. cit.
39. Finlay L. Through the looking glass: intersubjectivity and hermeneutic reflection. In: Finlay L and Gough B, editors. *Reflexivity: A Practical Guide for Researchers in Health and Social Sciences*. Oxford: Blackwell Science, 2003, 105–19.
40. Schon DA. *Educating the Reflective Practitioner*. San Francisco, CA: Jossey-Bass, 1987.
41. Johns C. *Becoming a Reflective Practitioner*. Oxford: Blackwell Science, 2000.
42. Finlay, op. cit.
43. Schon, op. cit.
44. Johns, op. cit.
45. Finlay, op. cit.
46. Kvale and Brickmann, op. cit.
47. MacMillan K. The next turn: reflexively analysing reflexive research. In: Finlay L and Gough B, editors. *Reflexivity: A Practical Guide for Researchers in Health and Social Sciences*. Oxford: Blackwell Science, 2003, 231–50.
48. Jasper M. Using reflective writing in research. *Journal of Research in Nursing*. 2005; **10**(3): 247–60.
49. Alaszewski A. *Using Diaries for Social Research*. London: Sage, 2006.
50. Koch T. Implementation of hermeneutic inquiry in nursing; philosophy, rigour and representation. *Journal of Advanced Nursing*. 1996; **24**: 174–84.
51. Trnobranski P. The decision to prolong life: ethical perspectives of a clinical dilemma. *Journal of Clinical Nursing*. 1996; **5**(4): 233–40.
52. Kvale and Brickmann, op. cit.

53. Mitchell D. An existential view: doing and being – the therapeutic relationship. In: Greenstreet W, editor. *Integrating Spirituality into Health and Social Care: Perspectives and Practical Approaches*. Oxford: Radcliffe Publishing, 2006, 111–13.

54. Punch KF. *Developing Effective Research Proposals*. London: Sage, 2006.

55. Schwandt TA. Three epistemological stances for qualitative inquiry. In: Denzin N and Lincoln YS, editors. *The Landscape of Qualitative Research: Theories and Issues*. Thousand Oaks, CA: Sage, 2003, 292–331.

56. Ibid.

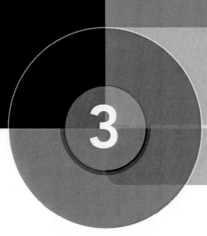

An outline of what was already known

3

The researcher comes to a study with a background that has evolved from their personal history and culture. In Heideggerian phenomenology this is described as a fore-structure of understanding.[1] Fore-structure is threefold in nature. First, fore-having is related to familiarity with the phenomenon that is the subject of study, which makes an interpretation possible. The second is fore-sight, which is the point of view generated by the researcher's background, from which an interpretation is made; and last comes fore-conception, where the researcher's experience may contribute to some anticipated expectation of interpretation.

Familiarity may result in aspects of understanding being taken for granted and therefore the researcher may lose sight of how fore-structure affects their interpretation of, and reflexive response to, research participants' disclosure. Hence it is important that a reflection on fore-structure precedes data collection to counteract any such oversight. Consequently, in this chapter I present an account of my scholarship, and a literature review that reflects my knowledge and understanding of spirituality and loss prior to commencement of the study.

My scholarship contributes to fore-structure, in that it encompasses exploration of, and publication on, both spirituality and loss in healthcare contexts, including why[2] and how[3] to teach loss to health and social care students, and pain;[4] curriculum development in palliative care;[5] literature review of teaching spirituality;[6] spirituality in organizations;[7] and contemporary discourse in spirituality.[8] A decade of experience in teaching spirituality culminated in my authoring/editing a reader, which reflects my thoughts on integration of spirituality in health and social care practice.[9]

The literature review that follows provides a synopsis of my fore-having and my familiarity with the phenomenon of loss and spirituality as a perspective of healthcare. This is explored within a number of themes, the first of which is the impact of loss on personal identity. Also, my understanding of spirituality as an aspect of being a person is considered, as is differentiation between spirituality and religion. The themes of meaning and purpose in life, forgiveness, relationship and hope are addressed in terms of spiritual need. The final theme gives some account of the cultural perspective of spirituality. This literature review also accounts for the remaining facets of fore-structure in reflecting my fore-sight, in linking spirituality with loss in healthcare contexts, and my fore-conception, in anticipating that this link is related to coping.

IMPACT OF LOSS ON PERSONAL IDENTITY

Chronic or terminal illness can undermine an individual's sense of identity. Whether abrupt or insidious in onset, the long-standing duration of illness that is managed rather than cured means that the chronically and terminally ill may benefit from support in facing the consequent challenges of their condition. A greater understanding of the processes used by nurses to help patients make sense of their situation could potentially enable nurses to facilitate the most effective support for those in their care.

Neimeyer,[10] a professor of psychology, well published in issues of chronic loss associated with dying and death, uses case studies to illustrate a critique of traditional theories and their descriptive stages of adaptation to loss. He proposes an alternative understanding, a constructivist approach founded on the assumption that reconstructing a world of meaning is central to the experience of grieving. The personal reality of loss is individual and not universal; it involves actively facing the challenges of loss rather than remaining passive. Personal meanings, not only of the loss itself, but also in relation to emotional, behavioural and physical responses, provide a holistic portrayal of adaptation to loss, rather than the more traditional focus on emotional reaction. In this way, significant loss is seen to transform an individual's world rather than lead to the recovery of a previous norm. Interestingly, Parkes'[11] studies from a psychiatric perspective of grief in adult life, first published in 1972, reflect what is currently regarded as traditional theory, describing a model of grief constituting four phases: shock, searching, despair and then adjustment. However, this is a rather narrow interpretation of his work on bereavement, given that he describes not only potential alarm and anger as a trauma response to loss and searching as a grief response, but also psycho-social transition as a process of adaptation to change, which involves the adoption of a new model of the world. Parkes[12] draws together ideas from research on stress, loss and crisis to propose psycho-social transition as a new conceptual field. This concept is still included in contemporary published work,[13] and although using different terminology, appears to have much in common with Neimeyer's[14] perspective above. Fundamentally, they convey the sense of us each creating an assumed world by organizing who we are, our identities, as we make sense of the self and the world by creating personal interpretations of our experiences. Consequently, when circumstances involving significant and permanent loss shake this sense of self and world, we try to interpret events in ways consistent with our identity and the ways in which we have understood past experience. Involvement with patients with terminal and chronic illness who struggle with their sense of identity in the face of life-changing events may trigger existential questioning by nurses that results in a shift in their assumed world. Raising the question 'why?' often reflects a search for existential meaning within particular life events that happen during the course of work. Such questioning is at the heart of what is meant by the term 'spiritual'.[15]

SPIRITUALITY AS AN INTEGRAL ASPECT OF EVERY PERSON

Historically, in Western society, nursing care was delivered within religious orders.[16] Every person was thought to have a spiritual potential and an awareness of, and relationship with, God that they would look to in order to make sense of their suffering, confirm some enduring value in themselves and above all find some meaning in their existence.[17] Attempts to move towards provision of secular care resulted in a fall in standards, for example the provision for the sick within the Elizabethan poor laws. The Enlightenment moved eighteenth-century society towards secularization and persons were viewed more analytically as comprising body, mind and spirit, rather than as an indivisible whole. By the nineteenth century a rising population and changes in medical knowledge meant that religious orders could no longer cope with the provision of nursing.[18] Florence Nightingale's middle-class status gave the role of the nurse a new respectability, providing the humanist philanthropist with a vocation previously associated with the religious. Although Nightingale did not require that nurses practise a religion, selection of those considered suitable to nurse was based on Judeo-Christian ethics and morals.[19] Nightingale's model of nursing embraced the humanity of persons in being 'covenantal',[20] in that nursing involved experiential knowing, often shared non-verbally within the nurse–patient relationship. Nursing action based on these shared moments unfolds as a transformative act that honours the art of nursing and the nurses' personal commitment to care.[21] However, the secularization of nursing continued and registration and moves towards professionalization as the twentieth century progressed moved nursing into contractual care, in line with task accomplishment values of an industrialized society.[22] While medical treatment of persons' physical disease gathered kudos, psychiatric care of persons' disease of the mind was relegated to second place, while the spiritual care of persons was difficult to find and, at best, something for the attention of chaplains and 'people like that'.[23]

The later part of the twentieth century saw a revival of interest in covenantal models of care, particularly in the work of Cicely Saunders[24] at St Christopher's Hospice, where the concept of caring for the whole person, or holistic care, reinvigorated an interest in the spiritual needs of persons, as well as managing their physical, social and psychological needs. Increasingly, nursing's professional and statutory bodies have formally affirmed the significance of spirituality. The Royal College of Nursing,[25] for example, has described spirituality as an integral aspect of the whole person. Similarly, it is increasingly featured in national health policy guidelines; for example, both the Department of Health[26] and the National Institute for Clinical Excellence[27] have acknowledged spiritual care as important within service provision.

Spirituality is a complex concept. Bradshaw[28] exemplifies this in her critique of the Royal College's standard on palliative nursing related to spiritual support. She challenges the implied dualism of spiritual care as a separate topic of care and prefers to describe spiritual care in nursing as an attempt to establish the nature of humanity. Her concern is that academic account of this concept is piecemeal and used to justify clinical care, rather than help nursing engage with the complexities of humanity. She proposes that spiritual care should not be the self-conscious delivery of an additional aspect of care but that compassionate care of the person is in itself the expression of spiritual care. However, the theologian Henri Nouwen[29] explains how compassion competes with our desire to 'do' something in the face of suffering:

Let us not underestimate how hard it is to listen and to be compassionate. Compassion is hard because it requires the inner disposition to go with others to the place where they are weak, vulnerable, lonely and broken. But this is not our spontaneous response to suffering. What we desire most is to do away with suffering by fleeing from it or finding a quick cure for it. As busy, active, relevant people, we want to earn our bread by making a real contribution. This means first and foremost doing something to show that our presence makes a difference. And so we ignore our greatest gift, which is our ability to be there, to listen and enter into solidarity with those who suffer (p. 34).

Regardless of debate, both health policy and contemporary models of nursing care agree that all persons have a spiritual dimension. Hence spiritual care needs to be addressed for the agnostic or atheist as well as for those with a religious affiliation.[30]

Comprehensive review of published literature and research demonstrates that spirituality cannot be conveyed in a single definition.[31,32] Some emphasize the qualitative benefit of fulfilment in the transcendent nature of spirituality as an essential part of wholeness, rather than entire dependence on the everyday world of the material.[33,34] Others, such as Burkhardt,[35] found on analysis of case studies what she described as an 'unfolding mystery' equated with the renewal that emerged following hardship or suffering. This renewal was sourced from an inner strength associated with inward reflection, supportive relationships, a sense of knowing self, closeness to nature and with a 'higher' being, all of which contributed to a feeling of harmony. This inner strength is reflected in the writings of the philosophical theologian, Paul Tillich,[36,37] whose perspective on spirituality encouraged 'God' to be seen as the depth, or ground, of all being, rather than reducing God to 'a being'.[38,39] In this way, Tillich argued, there can be no non-believers. This further affirms the spiritual dimension of all humanity, but it is in the individual's definition of 'God' that the true key to understanding spirituality is to be found. This is exemplified in Scherer's[40] description of spirituality in popular culture, where the rituals and symbols among sports supporters display characteristics of a secular religion outside of any understanding of 'God' as conceived by Tillich.

Burnard[41] points out that people cannot simply be divided into 'believers' and 'unbelievers', because fundamentally many people give little thought to spiritual issues. Writing as a nurse educationalist, he goes on to emphasize the importance of nurses clarifying their own belief and value systems before they are able to help patients with existential or 'ultimate' questions. Similarly, findings of a large-scale empirical study concerning spiritual pain at the end of life also advocated a greater awareness among caregivers of their own spiritual experiences.[42] The reason given for this is related to the human potential for vulnerability. In order to stay with all that is vulnerable in another person and support them in their need for spiritual care, we need to care for ourselves, to be aware of our own spirituality as a resource in coping with our own vulnerability. Clarity will also help us differentiate our needs from another's, and in so doing reduce the possibility of projecting our needs into another's situation.[43]

DIFFERENTIATING BETWEEN RELIGION AND SPIRITUALITY

Sheldrake[44] explores the history of the term 'spirituality'. Seated in Christian religion, the term seeks to express 'life in the spirit', the conscious human response to God that is both personal and ecclesial. He outlines changes in the meaning of spirituality that have emerged in Western Christianity in the later part of the twentieth century. These include the suggestion that spirituality is not exclusive to any particular Christian tradition, or necessarily with Christianity as a whole. Also, spirituality is not so much about perfection, but more to do with the complexity of human growth in the context of a living relationship with what is considered the 'Absolute'. In addition, spirituality is not limited to a concern with the interior life, but seeks an integration of all aspects of human life and experience. The broadening use of this term has contributed to its current relevance to, and use in, non-religious contexts.

Bradshaw's[45] research concerning the spiritual dimension is an exercise in concept analysis and clarification. Theology is used to clarify and explain, and critical reasoning to interpret, this concept. Philosophy is used as methodology, rather than either of the more conventional qualitative or quantitative approaches. Using a rational analysis of how things appear to be generates an understanding of reality, truth and meaning. The study analysis is comprehensive, but as McFarlane[46] points out, this research is a difficult read as it draws heavily on philosophical and theological vocabularies. Bradshaw[47] writes of how those freed from self-preoccupation by their knowledge of God's love were enabled to help others as an instrument of the love by which they themselves lived. This perspective reflects the historical roots of nursing as a religious vocation. The emphasis was on spiritual rather than physical care; support rather than cure. It is therefore not surprising that spirituality has often mistakenly been equated with religion by nurses.

However, Cicely Saunders,[48] a nurse, almoner and physician, and the founder of the modern hospice movement, was very clear in her differentiation between the two concepts. She believed spirituality was the wider concept and concerned moral values throughout life, and so memories, for example those that engendered guilt, were not necessarily seen in religious terms and consequently not relieved by religious rituals.

Heriot[49] reviewed literature and research concerned with spirituality and ageing. She also differentiates between religion and spirituality, and in doing so brings many of the dimensions of spirituality together. Spirituality is described as a broader notion, an umbrella under which religion and the needs of human spirit are found. Spirituality is described as being concerned with the personal interpretation of life and the inner resources of people, whereas religion is seen as an external, formal system of beliefs. Therefore, although spirituality is not synonymous with religion, for those who have a faith, religion is one means of fulfilling spiritual need.

A descriptive survey of cancer patients' spiritual coping strategies by Sodestrom and Martinson[50] found that the majority of patients exercised religious faith through spiritual activities such as praying as one means of coping. Later research by Fehring et al.[51] also found that religion was a means of coping for cancer patients, but their findings were more discerning in accounting for why religion helped. They differentiate between those patients who took their religion seriously and practised their faith as part of their daily lives, and those who participated in religious practice as a means of sociability, security or solace. The former are described as intrinsically religious and their faith provided psychic strength, meaning, purpose and transcendence as ways of coping. The latter are described as extrinsically religious and they draw on their religious group for social support to help them cope.

In her review of nursing literature that scanned 26 years, Emblem's[52] analysis found six words repeatedly appeared in definitions of religion. The definition that results from collating these describes religion as a person's organised system of beliefs, practices and form of worship. Consequently, for nurses who can relate to these systems, their religion may constitute a personal resource in helping them to cope with caring for the terminally or chronically ill. Religion may provide answers to existential questions of meaning related to the circumstances they find themselves in, or perhaps provide solace within a supportive social network. Similarly, nurses who do not have a religious faith may still draw on their own personal interpretation of life that constitutes their source of strength when faced with such questions, or their social network when needing solace.

SPIRITUAL NEEDS

Following a review of palliative literature Kellehear[53] defines spiritual need as seeking and finding meaning, transcending hardship and suffering. This is supported by wider reviews of published literature[54,55] where common themes of meaning and purpose, the need for fulfilling relationships, hope and forgiveness, emerge as spiritual needs, all of which are reflected in Kellehear's[56] theoretical model of spiritual needs in palliative care.

MEANING AND PURPOSE IN LIFE

The search for life's meaning and purpose, and the significance of existence, are frequently discussed in literature describing spirituality.[57,58] McColl[59] describes the relationship between spirituality and meaning as reciprocal, in that spirituality invests activities with meaning and meaningful activities express spirituality. The religious believer may understand the meaning and purpose of life as a mission, the source and taskmaster of this mission being God.[60] The meaning and purpose of life for non-believers may be a career, family, money or even self.[61,62] Frankl's[63] observation and experience of suffering in Nazi concentration camps resulted in his belief that an important determinant of survival of difficult circumstances is a sense of meaning and purpose in life that transcends the immediate situation.

Caring for others who are struggling to find meaning in their situations of loss requires personal vigilance on the part of the nurse. Wakefield[64] describes a case study of a patient she had nursed to illustrate nurses' inclination to protect themselves from the distress associated with a dying patient. She points out the inevitable sense of loss, and that relentless self-care needs to be an important feature of end of life care nursing. The suggested means of achieving this is to act out the advice given to bereaved relatives. This involves the nurse saying goodbye to the dead person as a form of social closure of caring interaction. Other suggestions involved sharing feelings through stories, reflection and debriefing, as well as asking any questions that may help them make sense of events. In this way, nurses' personal vigilance maintains their own emotional and spiritual capacity to deal with patients' and their relatives' losses.[65]

FORGIVENESS

Stanworth[66] describes spirituality as more easily recognised than explained. Using metaphor she describes the spiritual dimension as a horizon that is further away, broader and more ungraspable than any other. In glimpsing this ultimate horizon the foreground is not changed, but its meaning can be radically altered. She goes on to explain that in the same way, past events cannot be altered, but can be seen in a fresh light, and this change is the experience of forgiveness. In end of life care situations, guilt due to a sense of failing to live up to expectations can be a cause of spiritual distress.[67] Attentive nurses may recognize the nature of this distress and facilitate the means for patients to achieve a need to forgive or be forgiven.

McCullough et al.[68] propose that forgiveness involves constructive psychological change toward a transgression, and that this change takes time. The ways in which individuals appraise transgressions impact their ability to forgive.[69] Attributional theorists emphasize the influence of the degree of responsibility or blame attributed for the transgression, as opposed to interdependence theorists, who emphasize the role of relationship commitment. Others emphasize the effect of empathic emotions that stimulate helping behaviour due to, for example, a desire to restore a breached relationship. Following their own study, McCullough et al.[70] propose an additional aptitude that facilitates forgiveness. The study sample was large, involving 213 women and 91 men representing a variety of cultural and ethnic backgrounds. Participants were undergraduates and so the mean age was low at just over 19 years. Participants completed an initial questionnaire identifying an occasion when they had been hurt or offended and a final questionnaire about their current feelings related to this event, but in between they completed a writing task where one third wrote about the benefits that had come out of this event, one third about the traumatic features and the remaining third wrote about a topic other than the event. McCullough *et al.*[71] found that the ability to focus on the benefits gained from a transgression, such as realization of personal inner strength or renewed spirituality, helps negate some of the psychological costs, such as loss of trust, and so enables forgiveness.

Clearly, the mean age of patients in end of life situations exceeds that of participants in McCullough *et al.*'s[72] study. However, the principle that the way in which individuals appraise transgressions impacts their ability to forgive is corroborated in published comment that describes practice experience, such as Saunders[73] below. Given that unforgiveness is itself a cause of stress due to the nature of the emotions generated, the ability to replace negative emotions such as anger with positive emotions such as empathy means that forgiveness provides a means of coping.[74] The capacity to forgive oneself, to shift emotional appraisal from negative to positive, or as Myco[75] suggests, to live with one's flaws, is reflected in the experience of Saunders'[76] work with dying patients:

There is a progression from trust in the acceptance by others of all the things in ourselves that we regret into a faith in forgiveness, where we at last believe that they have no more power to hurt us or anyone else. We cannot alter what has happened or what we have done, but we can come to believe that the meaning of the past can be changed. From this comes an ability to forgive ourselves. This may never be expressed in words on either side but the quality of the ensuing peace is unmistakable. (Cicely Saunders. *Living With Dying: a Guide to Palliative Care*. 3rd ed. 1995, 55. By permission of Oxford University Press.)

Stanworth[77] illustrates Saunders'[78] point. She recounts how a middle-aged woman who was paralysed by motor neurone disease explains how her feelings of guilt for being divorced twice are disappearing. She describes how her illness has helped her see things in a new perspective. She feels her sense of freedom is evident in her poems and has learned to love people for what they are. She tells of how her illness has seen her relinquish anger and unhappiness and set her on a path to peaceful calm.

A search for meaning is often evidenced by existential questioning, asking 'why'? There is often no known answer to existential questions that patients pose, and consequently nurses should not burden themselves with guilt when they are unable to respond or understand.

RELATIONSHIPS

Relationships signify another spiritual need, whether with others, a transcendent power or the natural environment. The nature of love given and received within relationships is seen to differ. Literature suggests human love is conditional, dependent on 'if' the other satisfies a need, or 'because' of what the other has, who they are and what they are,[79,80] or dependent on the attractive qualities of others.[81] This is contrasted with unconditional love, usually associated with a 'higher power' or God. Unconditional love is described in various ways, as a gift, selfless, gracious, undemanding[82] and self-giving love.[83]

However, Campbell[84] proposes a theology of professional care in which he refers to professionals having the potential to give 'moderated' love, which is unconditional. This moderated love appears synonymous with Nightingale's[85] view of care as covenantal, being concerned as much with 'how' care is given as with what is 'done'.[86] The relationship between patient and nurse in covenantal care is one of mutual sharing, freely given as part of personal commitment.[87]

Campbell[88] describes the sharing of self in a professional context, in order to enhance care, as an example of self-transcendence.

The terminally and chronically ill may well have long-term healthcare needs that result in nurses coming to know their patients and their carers very well. The challenge for professionals in sharing self is that they risk suffering grief following the loss of those they care for. A study by McIntyre[89] that involved interviewing 16 nursing staff from eight wards, exemplified how nurses 'grieve too' when they care for the dying and their relatives. An earlier study by Davies and Oberle[90] involved comparative analysis of data derived from in-depth, retrospective descriptions of the care given by a supportive care nurse to 10 palliative care patients and their relatives. They found that valuing the inherent worth of others, and in particular of individual patients she came to know, was a key concept related to the nurse as a person, as was preserving her own integrity. The latter was achieved partly by the nurse's ability to maintain feelings of self-worth and self-esteem by periodic reflection on meaning in relation to the work she was doing, feedback from others that contributed to her feeling that she made a difference, continual self-assessment of whether she was doing the right things for the right reason, and acknowledging and accepting her own feelings, including those of grief. In addition, integrity was sustained by maintaining energy levels. This was achieved by setting limits, using strategies of distancing to regain control, using humour, hiding personal feelings, learning from mistakes and sharing frustrations. Although focused on a single nurse's experiences, this study hones in on the vital issue of nurses needing to maintain their own integrity if they are to continue to help end of life care patients and their families.

HOPE

The concept of hope is an integral aspect of human spirituality. It concerns a sense of future and is described by Bauckham and Hart[91] as sourced from our capacity to imagine otherwise, our potential to transcend any shortfall or challenges in our current circumstances, and hope for something better than the present affords.

Desroche's[92] description of hope reflects both its intangibility and its potential irrationality. He uses myth as the setting, and compares hope to a rope thrown in the air, anchored in cloud and able to carry the weight of the man that climbs it. This description is also symbolic, in reflecting our human tendency to cling onto hope in life's most difficult moments.[93]

Nurses may have difficulty in conveying hope in an extremely disabling disorder, such as motor neurone disease,[94] or appear pessimistic to avoid giving false hope.[95] There are a number of studies available that explore hope. These potentially raise nurses' awareness of strategies that may enhance hope, both for themselves and for those they care for in practice, for instance an American study by Herth.[96] This used a convenience sample of 30 terminally ill adults accessing support from three hospices, each patient having a prognosis of six months or less. Patient semi-structured interviews, together with responses to a hope index tool and background information, allowed triangulation of cross-sectional data. In addition, 10 patients were interviewed and completed the hope index tool on two further occasions: first when impairment of their ability to complete activities of daily living became severe, and then when signs and symptoms indicated that they were likely to die within two weeks. Extraordinarily, the published account of this research makes no mention of the ethical significance of repeated access to participants who are dying, in utilizing their 'time left' to live, nor does it acknowledge the changing nature of end-stage illness in relation to participants' ability to continue to contribute. The study was replicated in England by Buckley and Herth,[97] and on this occasion ethical considerations were acknowledged. This second study supported the findings of the first in that hope remained present despite nearness to death, as well as corroborating that interpersonal connectedness, spiritual base, attainable aims, affirmation of worth, lightheartedness, personal attributes and uplifting memories all provided ways in which hope could be fostered.

These studies provide a potentially useful guide in maintaining and inspiring hope in those needing to focus particularly on 'being' in the present moment. The strategies work on the premise that giving up on particular hopes does not mean giving up on hope altogether.[98] They are as beneficial for the nurse as their patient in that they help nurses locate hope in caring for the terminally ill. Nurses hope to facilitate a 'good' death by allowing patients and their family to express their preferences, and exercise control of events during their care.[99]

Interpersonal connectedness is one means of fostering hope, and is described by Buckley and Herth[100] as comprising meaningful relationships, of being loved and giving love. Acknowledging the universal nature of hope may be the first step in enabling professional carers to make interpersonal connections with those in their care. Having a sense of something that is important to all humanity could provide some common ground on which to start building a therapeutic relationship. The study by Davies and Oberle[101] illustrates that a nurse providing supportive and palliative care 'globally' valued the inherent worth of others, regardless of individual characteristics, and then, in connecting with the patient and family, developing a rapport and establishing trust, she came to value the patient and family in a more 'particular', individualized way. Similarly, in her study which considered nursing interventions for engendering hope in the chronically and terminally ill, Herth[102] found that connectedness was rated highly by professionals.

Uplifting memories also fostered hope; in having a temporal dimension, the patient's past is reflected on in the present, and contributes to hope in its association with the future. Relationships that are open to sharing these moments of reflection provide opportunities to affirm mutual worth. Buckley and Herth[103] found patients shared good memories that seemed to be important to hope. They found attitudes of staff important in helping patients remain hopeful. Patients particularly valued the 'little things' that staff 'bothered' to find out for them. Similarly, hope was fostered by personal attributes or characteristics such as optimism and cheerfulness, which, if nurtured, provide opportunity for lightheartedness. Spontaneity, sensitivity in the use of humour and the ability to laugh as the moment dictates create joyous moments for both patient and professional that can contribute to sustaining hope.[104,105]

In Morse and Doberneck's[106] qualitative study describing the concept of hope, interview data was gathered from four participant groups, which included patients with chronic illness (heart disease) and disability (spinal cord injury). Concept analysis was thorough, starting with identification of processes or characteristics of hope (abstract components) from a single account that provided the best example illustrating hope. These abstract components represented a tentative framework constituting the concept. Choosing the 'best example account' initially appears to be subject to researcher bias, however, this choice is 'tested' by finding examples of identified components of hope in other accounts. If this search proved fruitless, the original characteristics were wrong, and the process was repeated using another example account. Finally, data from each group interviewed was compared component by component. Findings identified seven attributes or components. First, hope is a response to a threat that results in a plan, a goal to resolve the problem. An awareness of the significance, the cost of not achieving the goal motivates planning to make it a reality. This involves assessment, selection and utilization of resources, both internal and external, together with any support that will help the achievement of the goal. Lastly, the plan to reach the goal is re-evaluated and revised in the throes of striving to reach the goal. Collectively, these seven attributes or components create a markedly goal-oriented description of the concept of hope.

Some findings in this study were similar to those of Buckley and Herth,[107] for example in relation to hope and relationships. Morse and Doberneck[108] found that the attainment of a goal is not achieved alone, but includes the solicitation of mutually supportive relationships. These relationships are balanced, and so it is rare for all members to have doubts about the feasibility of a goal at the same time. Support strategies used in these relationships may be hands-on support, or indirect support that bolsters the individual's ability to deal with their situation, for example affirming personal attributes such as courage or endurance.[109] Nurses are party to these mutually supportive relationships.

SPIRITUALITY AND CULTURE

Spirituality reflects socio-cultural values.[110] Different cultures vary in their philosophical stances. The Western transcendent view of spirituality supports the concept of a reality beyond the material world.[111] Spirit is localized in time and place within individual consciousness, as that part concerned with ultimate awareness, meaning, value and purpose.[112] In contrast, Eastern pantheism views the world as a single entity, spirituality being synonymous with the forces of nature.[113] The emphasis is on spirit as a non-local quality, timeless, spaceless, and an immortal element that links humanity with the environment and, ultimately, the universe.[114]

Garner[115] considers the secularization of Western societies as culturally in-built, in that there is a refusal to believe that God can be heard, and consequently no steps are taken to hear. Jarvis[116] sees the absence of metaphysical or supernatural belief, together with an inability by many to understand the complexities of science and technology, as constituting socio-cultural systems that contribute to a void in contemporary society, a lack of meaning in our material world. This lack of meaning appears to have triggered what Tacey[117] describes as a counter-cultural revolution, one of spirituality that finds the sacred everywhere, a direct political and philosophical challenge to traditional notions of sacredness such as the body, nature, the feminine and the physical environment.

Heelas and Woodhead[118] describe the 'subjective turn' as a major cultural shift. Rather than a life determined by duty, obligation or role, this cultural shift reflects a life centred more on an individual's subjective experience. In this way, the individual becomes their own authority, rather than deferring to a higher authority. Postmodern individualism is certainly reflected in the shift from professional paternalism to increasing autonomy for those accessing healthcare services.[119] The language of the subjective turn is used by Heelas and Woodhead,[120] to distinguish between religion and spirituality. Religion is thought to subordinate life to a higher authority associated with transcendent meaning, whereas the subjective life, associated with spirituality, is thought to cultivate what is unique and sacred within individuals. Their research considered religion and spirituality in a town in North East England. The primary aim was to establish the numerical significance of 'alternative spirituality' or 'the holistic milieu' taking place outside broader institutional contexts such as hospitals. Results reflected unequivocal evidence of growth in alternative spirituality, which in their study constituted complementary and alternative medicine.

However, contemporary discourse on nursing spirituality in a secularized society can potentially create greater confusion rather than further clarity.[121] Heelas[122] later goes on to make a theoretical argument that equates nursing spirituality with complementary and alternative therapy, described as 'holistic spirituality'. Nurses, as members of contemporary society, share the values and beliefs of the culture in which they have been educated, live and work. It is not unreasonable to support the view that the increased interest in complementary and alternative medicine is reflected among nurses, but not necessarily in their contracts of employment. However, they may be involved in the practice of referral of patients to alternative and complementary therapists as part of healthcare provision. It is important that the myth sourced from nursing's religious roots, equating spirituality with religious belief and practice, is not replaced with a new myth, sourced from nurses' current secular cultural roots, that spirituality equates with a belief in complementary and alternative medical practice.[123] There are a number of significant differences between Heelas'[124] theoretical account of holistic spirituality and nursing research and literature that addresses spirituality as a perspective of holistic care. Comparison of these discourses demonstrates that spirituality as a perspective of holistic care is a more comprehensive discourse, within which holistic spirituality, as described by Heelas,[125] reflects an option for providing spiritual care.[126]

McGrath[127] suggests that we do not have limitless possibilities of ways to act, or an infinite number of theories concerning existence, and that culture is the template that outlines what the possibilities are. She also describes the medical model of care as a cultural system that nurses are very familiar with, emphasising disease and fact over experience and belief. This therefore tends to limit nurses to an approach that reduces care to a concern with task and function. McGrath[128] proposes that conceptualising illness as a problem of meaning is an alternative approach that offers a way of understanding the role of culture in framing behaviour and belief. In this way, McGrath[129] links cultural and spiritual care, and encourages professionals to reflect on the ways they approach and respond to patients with chronic and terminal illness. Nurses, therefore, need to consider their own beliefs and behaviours around terminal and chronic illness, as well as their skills in sensitive questioning and active listening. Although it is important for nurses to continue 'doing' care for those with physical and pathological disorders, McGrath's suggestion encourages nurses to consider their style of approach to patients, 'how' they are with those in their care.

Friedemann[130] developed a framework of systemic organization to serve as a theoretical basis for family nursing. This was later applied to nursing the spirit,[131] and is useful in conveying an understanding of a number of emotions and behaviours displayed by patients and their relatives in end of life care situations. Friedemann[132] claims that the ideal condition of all systems is one of 'congruence' or harmony, but as all systems are subject to change and conflicting values, congruence is never reached. The consequent tension is experienced as anxiety. Friedemann et al.[133] link culture to the way in which individuals manage the anxiety that results from a change in health status. They believe that humans are equipped to buffer the effect of the tension that such changes bring by balancing control in their lives with spirituality. The ideal balance is individually determined, depending on the emphasis that culture, beliefs and values place on either control or spirituality. In a Western culture, which predominantly values control, individuals tend to strive to re-establish pre-existing conditions. This involves deliberate behavioural strategies such as seeking medical treatment for illnesses. Nurses are involved in both the care and treatment of illness, for example in the administration of prescribed medication. Control is not always possible. The sense of loss of control may result in a variety of emotions on the patient's or relative's part, such as anxiety, anger and resentment. These emotions may be directed at nurses at a time when professional carers are also coping with similar emotions in facing their own inability to control the outcome of care.

Friedemann et al.[134] suggest an increased emphasis on spirituality allows a more philosophical approach, which facilitates transcending the immediate situation and so helps in acceptance of the limits of human control on the natural order of events. Consequently, spirituality as an alternative resource to control provides a defence against anxiety and is particularly appropriate where change, such as terminal or chronic illness, is not reversible. Similarly, spirituality may allow the nurses to transcend their immediate environment, to see their situation in a wider perspective, one that is outside the artificial limits of control. In this way, nurses may be less anxious, and possibly better able to deliver supportive care.

SUMMARY

This account of fore-structure of understanding provides an overview of the knowledge and experience that has brought me to this study's particular focus: on spirituality as a resource in coping with loss. Publications that have been the product of my scholarship in both spirituality and loss provide evidence of comprehensive literature search in both subjects as a constituent element of my knowledge.

The purpose of my account of fore-structure of understanding, from a phenomenological perspective, is one of transparency, to reflect a subjective self-awareness which acknowledges that what I know impacts how I interpret participants' descriptions of their experience. This reflexivity allows critique of assumptions I have made, and an awareness of how they are changed in the throes of interview, or on analysis of interview transcripts. Conscious self-awareness is promoted further by my keeping an account of my reflective thoughts throughout the study, but particularly in relation to data collection and analysis.

My knowledge and experience have illuminated how elusive defining spirituality is, and how difficult this concept is to describe. It is both covert, in constituting the core of self, and overt, reflected in the way we live, in what we do, and how we 'are' with others. Published literature and policy guidelines imply that spirituality is a resource for coping with loss but offer little understanding in identifying how nurses use spirituality to help them care for patients facing life-threatening illness. This study addresses these issues.

REFERENCES

1. Plager KA. Hermeneutic phenomenology: a method for family health and health promotion study in nursing. In: Benner P, editor. *Interpretative Phenomenology*. Thousand Oaks, CA: Sage, 1994, 65–83.
2. Greenstreet W. Why nurses need to understand the principles of bereavement theory. *British Journal of Nursing*. 2004; **13**(10): 590–3.
3. Greenstreet W. Loss, grief and bereavement in interprofessional education, an example of process: anecdotes and accounts. *Nurse Education in Practice*. 2005; **5**: 281–8.
4. Greenstreet W. The concept of total pain: a focused patient care study. *British Journal of Nursing*. 2001; **10**(19): 1248–55.
5. Greenstreet W. Bridging the specialist-generalist divide: a creative Master's programme initiative. *International Journal of Palliative Nursing*. 2005; **11**(12): 638–42.
6. Greenstreet W. Teaching spirituality in nursing: a literature review. *Nurse Education Today*. 1999; **19**: 649–58.
7. Greenstreet W. Conference Report, Spirituality in organisations – exploring the way forward: International Conference on Organisational Spirituality. *Spirituality and Health International*. 2005; **6**(3): 176–7.
8. Greenstreet W. Synchronicity and dissonance: nursing, spirituality and contemporary discourse. *Spirituality and Health International*. 2007; **8**(2): 92–100.

9. Greenstreet W, editor. *Integrating Spirituality in Health and Social Care: Perspectives and Practical Approaches*. Oxford: Radcliffe Publishing, 2006.

10. Neimeyer RA. Meaning reconstruction and the experience of chronic loss. In: Doka KJ and Davidson J, editors. *Living With Grief When Illness is Prolonged*. Bristol: Taylor Francis, 1997, 159–76.

11. Parkes CM. *Bereavement, Studies of Grief in Adult Life*. 3rd ed. Routledge, London, 1996.

12. Parkes CM. Psycho-social transition: a field for study. *Social Science and Medicine*. 1971; **5**: 101–5.

13. Parkes CM. Bereavement as a psychosocial transition: processes of adaption to change. In: Dickinson D, Johnson J and Katz JS, editors. *Death, Dying and Bereavement*. London: Sage/Open University Press, 2000, 325–31.

14. Neimeyer, op. cit.

15. Speck P. Nursing the soul. *Nursing Times*. 1992; **88**(23): 22.

16. McGilloway O. Spiritual care: the potential for healing. In: McGilloway O and Myco F, editors. *Nursing and Spiritual Care*. London: Harper and Row, 1985, 74–84.

17. Pett D. The hospital chaplain. *Nursing Times*. 1973; **69**: 405–6.

18. Baly ME. (1980) *Nursing and Social Change*. London: Heinemann, 1980.

19. Widerquist JG. The spirituality of Florence Nightingale. *Nursing Research*. 1992; **41**(1): 49–55.

20. Bradshaw A. *Lighting the Lamp: the Spiritual Dimension of Nursing Care*. Harrow: Scutari Press, 1994.

21. Clements PT and Averill JB. Finding patterns of knowing in the work of Florence Nightingale. *Nursing Outlook*. 2006; **54**: 268–74.

22. Stuart EM, Dockro JP and Mandle CL. Spirituality in health and healing: a clinical program. *Holistic Nursing Practice*. 1989; **3**(3): 35–46.

23. McGilloway, op. cit.

24. Saunders C. Care for the dying. *Patient Care (UK)*. 1976; **III**: 6.

25. Royal College of Nursing. *Standards of Care: Palliative Nursing*. London: Royal College of Nursing, 1993.

26. Department of Health. *NHS Chaplaincy: Meeting the Religious and Spiritual Needs of Patients and Staff*. London: Department of Health, 2003.

27. National Institute for Clinical Excellence. *Supportive and Palliative Care for People with Cancer*: NICE Guidelines CSGSP. London: NICE, March 2004. www.nice.org.uk/guidance/csgsp

28. Bradshaw A. The legacy of Nightingale. *Nursing Times*. 1996; **92**(6): 42–3.

29. Nouwen H. *The Way of the Heart*. London: Harper, 1981.

30. Burnard P. Giving spiritual care. *Journal of Community Nursing*. 1993; **7**(1): 16–18.

31. Greenstreet, Teaching spirituality in nursing: a literature review, op. cit.

32. Greenstreet W. Clarifying the concept. In: Greenstreet W, editor. *Integrating Spirituality in Health and Social Care: Perspectives and Practical Approaches*. Oxford: Radcliffe Publishing, 2006, 7–19.

33. O'Brien ME. The need for spiritual integrity. In: Yura H and Walsh MB, editors. *Human Needs and the Nursing Process*. Norwalk, CT: Appleton-Century-Crofts, 1982, 85–115.

34. Hover-Kramer D. Creating a context for self healing: the transpersonal perspective. *Holistic Nursing Practice*. 1989; **3**(3): 27–34.

35. Burkhardt M A. Spirituality: an analysis of the concept. *Holistic Nursing Practice*. 1989; **3**(3): 69–77.

36. Tillich P. *The Protestant Era*. Translated by James Luther Adams. Chicago, IL: University of Chicago Press, 1948.
37. Tillich P. *The Courage to Be*. London: New Haven, 1953.
38. Thiselton AC. Tillich. In: Ferguson SB and Wright DF, editors. *New Dictionary of Theology*. Leicester: Inter-Varsity Press, 1988, 687–8.
39. Harrison J and Burnard P. *Spirituality and Nursing Practice*. Aldershot: Avenbury, 1993.
40. Scherer B. Faith and experience: paradigms of spirituality. In: Greenstreet W, editor. *Integrating Spirituality in Health and Social Care: Perspectives and Practical Approaches*. Oxford: Radcliffe Publishing, 2006, 89–100.
41. Burnard P. The spiritual needs of atheists and agnostics. *Professional Nurse*. 1988; December: 130–2.
42. Cornette K. For whenever I am weak, I am strong… *International Journal of Palliative Nursing*. 1997; **3** (1): 6–13.
43. Ibid.
44. Sheldrake P. *Spirituality and History*. London: SPCK, 1991.
45. Bradshaw, *Lighting the Lamp: the Spiritual Dimension of Nursing Care*, op. cit.
46. McFarlane J. Foreword. In: Bradshaw A. *Lighting the Lamp: the Spiritual Dimension of Nursing Care*. Harrow: Scutari Press, 1994, xxvii–xxxviii.
47. Bradshaw, *Lighting the Lamp: the Spiritual Dimension of Nursing Care*, op. cit.
48. Saunders C. Spiritual pain. *Journal of Palliative Care*. 1988; **4**(3): 30.
49. Heriot CS. Spirituality and ageing. *Holistic Nursing Practice*. 1992; **7**(1): 22–31.
50. Sodestrom KE and Martinson IM. Patients' spiritual coping strategies: a study of nurse and patient perspectives. *Oncology Nursing Forum*. 1987; **14**(2): 41–6.
51. Fehring RJ, Miller JF and Shaw C. Spiritual well–being, religiosity, hope, depression, and other mood states in elderly people coping with cancer. *Oncology Nursing Forum*. 1997; **24**(4): 663–71.
52. Emblen JD. Religion and spirituality defined according to current use in nursing literature. *Journal of Professional Nursing*. 1992; **8**(1): 41–7.
53. Kellehear A. Spirituality and palliative care: a model of needs. *Palliative Medicine*. 2000; **14**(2): 149–55.
54. Greenstreet. Teaching spirituality in nursing: a literature review, op. cit.
55. Greenstreet. Clarifying the concept, op. cit.
56. Kellehear, op. cit.
57. Martsolf D and Mickley J. The concept of spirituality in nursing theories: differing world-views and the extent of focus. *Journal of Advanced Nursing*. 1998; **27**(2): 294–303.
58. Narayanasamy A. Commentary. *Journal of Advanced Nursing*. 2004; **45**(5): 462–4.
59. McColl AM. Spirit, occupation and disability. *Canadian Journal of Occupational Therapy*. 2000; **67**(4): 217–28.
60. Fish S and Shelley JA. *Spiritual Care: the Nurse's Role*. Westmont, IL: InterVarsity Press, 1978.
61. Oldnall A. A critical analysis of nursing: meeting the spiritual needs of patients. *Journal of Advanced Nursing*. 1996; **23**: 138–44.
62. Harrison and Burnard, op. cit.
63. Frankl VE. *Man's Search for Meaning*. New York: Washington Square Press, 1984.
64. Wakefield A. Nurse responses to death and dying: a need for relentless self-care. *International Journal of Palliative Nursing*. 2000; **6**: 245–55.

65. Kinghorn S and Duncan F. Living with loss. In: Lugton J and McIntyre R, editors. *Palliative Care: The Nursing Role*. Edinburgh: Elsevier/Churchill Livingstone, 2005, 303–5.

66. Stanworth R. Attention: a potential vehicle for spiritual care. *Journal of Palliative Care*. 2002; **18**(3): 192–5.

67. Narayanasamy A. *Spiritual Care: A Practical Guide for Nurses and Health Care Professionals*. 2nd ed. Wiltshire: Quay, 2001.

68. McCullough ME, Fincham FD and Tsang JA. Forgiveness, forbearance, and time: the temporal unfolding of transgression-related interpersonal motivations. *Journal of Personality and Social Psychology*. 2003; **84**: 540–57.

69. McCullough ME, Root LM and Cohen AD. Writing about the benefits of an interpersonal transgression facilitates forgiveness. *Journal of Consulting and Clinical Psychology*. 2006; **74**(5): 887–97.

70. Ibid.

71. Ibid.

72. Ibid.

73. Saunders C. *Living with Dying: a Guide to Palliative Care*. 3rd ed. Oxford: Oxford University Press, 1995.

74. Davis DE, Worthington EL, Hook JN *et al*. Relational spirituality and the development of the similarity of the offender's spirituality scale. *Psychology of Religion and Spirituality*. 2009; **1**(4): 249–62.

75. Myco F. The non-believer in the health care situation. In McGilloway O and Myco F (eds) *Nursing and Spiritual Care*. London: Harper and Row, 1985, 36–52.

76. Saunders. *Living with Dying: a Guide to Palliative Care*, op. cit.

77. Stanworth R. When spiritual horizons beckon: recognizing ultimate meaning at the end of life. *Omega*. 2006; **15**(1–2): 27–38.

78. Saunders. *Living with Dying: a Guide to Palliative Care*, op. cit.

79. Lewis, CS. *The Four Loves*. Glasgow: Fontana, 1971.

80. Fish and Shelley, op. cit.

81. Bradshaw, *Lighting the Lamp: the Spiritual Dimension of Nursing Care*, op. cit.

82. Lewis, *The Four Loves*, op. cit.

83. Bradshaw, *Lighting the Lamp: the Spiritual Dimension of Nursing Care*, op. cit.

84. Campbell A. *Moderated Love: a Theology of Professional Care*. London: SPCK, 1984.

85. Nightingale F. *Notes on Nursing: What It Is and What It Is Not*. London: Butterworths, 1859.

86. Greenstreet. Synchronicity and dissonance: nursing, spirituality and contemporary discourse, op. cit.

87. Bradshaw. *Lighting the Lamp: the Spiritual Dimension of Nursing Care*, op. cit.

88. Campbell, op. cit.

89. McIntyre R. *Nursing Support for Families of Dying Patients*. London: Whurr, 2002.

90. Davies B and Oberle K. Dimensions of the supportive role of the nurse in palliative care. *Oncology Nursing Forum*. 1990; **17**(1): 87–94.

91. Bauckham R and Hart T. *Hope against Hope*. London: Darton, Longman and Todd, 1999.

92. Desroche H. *The Sociology of Hope*. London: Routledge & Kegan Paul, 1979.

93. Greenstreet W and Fiddian M. Sustaining hope. In: Greenstreet W, editor. *Integrating Spirituality in Health and Social Care: Perspectives and Practical Approaches*. Oxford: Radcliffe Publishing, 2006, 62–75.

94. Macleod R and Carter H. Health professionals' perception of hope: understanding its significance in the care of people who are dying. *Mortality*. 1999; **4**(3): 309–17.

95. Faulkner A and Maquire P. *Talking to Cancer Patients and Their Relatives*. Oxford: Oxford University Press, 1994.

96. Herth K. Fostering hope in terminally ill people. *Journal of Advanced Nursing*. 1990; **15**: 1250–9.

97. Buckley J and Herth K. Fostering hope in terminally ill people. *Nursing Standard*. 2004; **19**(10): 33–41.

98. Greenstreet and Fiddian, op. cit.

99. Seale C. What happens in hospices: a review of the literature. *Social Science and Medicine*. 1989; **28**(6): 551–9.

100. Buckley and Herth, op. cit.

101. Davies and Oberle, op. cit.

102. Herth K. Engendering hope in the chronically and terminally ill: nursing interventions. *American Journal of Hospice and Palliative Care*. 1995; **12**: 31–9.

103. Buckley and Herth, op. cit.

104. Herth. Fostering hope in terminally ill people, op. cit.

105. Buckley and Herth, op. cit.

106. Morse J and Doberneck B. Delineating the concept of hope. *Image: the Journal of Nursing Scholarship*. 1995; **27**(4): 227–85.

107. Buckley and Herth, op. cit.

108. Morse J and Doberneck B, op. cit.

109. Penrod J and Morse J. Strategies for assessing and fostering hope: the hope assessment guide. *Oncology Nursing Forum*. 1997; **24**(6): 1055–63.

110. Sheldrake, op. cit.

111. Bradshaw. *Lighting the Lamp: the Spiritual Dimension of Nursing Care*, op. cit.

112. O'Rawe Amenta M. Spiritual care: the heart of palliative nursing. *International Journal of Palliative Nursing*. 1997; **3**(1): 4.

113. Bradshaw. *Lighting the Lamp: the Spiritual Dimension of Nursing Care*, op. cit.

114. Heliker D. Re-evaluation of nursing diagnosis: spiritual distress. *Nursing Forum*. 1992; **27**(4): 15–20.

115. Garner C. What on earth is spirituality? In: Robson J and Lonsdale D, editors. *Can Spirituality be Taught?* Nottingham: Association of Centres of Adult Theological Association and British Council of Churches, 1987, 1–8.

116. Jarvis P. Meaning, being and learning. In: Jarvis P and Walters N, editors. *Adult Education and Theological Interpretations*. Malabar, FL: Krieger, 1993, 237–58.

117. Tacey D. *The Spirituality Revolution: the Emergence of Contemporary Spirituality*. Hove: Brunner Routledge, 2004.

118. Heelas P and Woodhead L. *The Spiritual Revolution: Why Religion Is Giving Way to Spirituality*. Oxford: Blackwell, 2005.

119. Greenstreet. Synchronicity and dissonance: nursing, spirituality and contemporary discourse, op. cit.

120. Heelas and Woodhead, op. cit.

121. Greenstreet. Synchronicity and dissonance: nursing, spirituality and contemporary discourse, op. cit.

122. Heelas P. Nursing spirituality. *Spirituality and Health International* (2006) **7**(1): 8–23.

123. Greenstreet. Synchronicity and dissonance: nursing, spirituality and contemporary discourse, op. cit.

124. Heelas, op. cit.

125. Ibid.

126. Greenstreet. Synchronicity and dissonance: nursing, spirituality and contemporary discourse, op. cit.

127. McGrath B. Illness as a problem of meaning: moving culture from the classroom to the clinic. *Advances in Nursing Science*. 1998; **21**(2): 17–29.

128. Ibid.

129. Ibid.

130. Friedemann M. *The Framework of Systemic Organization: A Conceptual Approach to Families and Nursing*. Thousand Oaks, CA: Sage, 1995.

131. Friedemann M, Mouch J and Racey T. Nursing the spirit: the framework of systemic organization. *Journal of Advanced Nursing*. 2002; **39**(4): 325–32.

132. Friedemann, op. cit.

133. Friedemann, Mouch and Racey. op. cit.

134. Ibid.

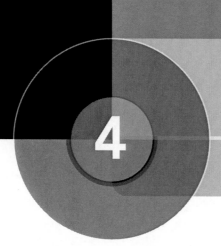

Involving nurses as research participants

The choice of method of data collection in any research project must always be one that provides data that addresses the focus of the study. For this reason, this chapter starts by revisiting the study's aims and objectives. The rationale for the choice of sampling research participants, the use of semi-structured interviews to collect data, ethical considerations for data collection and the value of maintaining a research diary have already been addressed (see Chapter 2). Therefore the main part of this chapter concerns the practicalities of accessing nurses as research participants and conducting semi-structured interviews as the primary means of collecting data.

AIM OF THE STUDY

The study aims to explore nurses' lived experience of spirituality as a means of helping patients to cope with loss associated with terminal or chronic disease.

OBJECTIVES OF THE STUDY

- To gain an understanding of nurses' perceptions of spirituality as an aspect of person-centred care.
- To explore the extent to which nurses facilitate spirituality as a source of coping.
- To explore how nurses use their personal resources in caring for those with chronic and terminal conditions.

ACCESSING NURSES TO PARTICIPATE

In purposively choosing nurses whose experience was likely to involve end of life care practice and so be impacted by issues of spirituality in situations of loss, my hope was that data would provide in-depth information[1] that would address the aim and objectives of the study. Therefore, when selecting practice environments for purposive sampling, exclusion criteria included acute settings, practice contexts where patient throughput is rapid and nurses working outside South East England.

Access to a hospice, care home and community primary care trust was negotiated and permission to carry out the study was sought from the senior nursing manager of each practice setting. Registered nurses with at least three years' experience in practice who were now working in the selected hospice, community primary care team and care home were invited to participate in a semi-structured interview. The sample reflected both a degree of heterogeneity, in that nurses were sourced from different practice settings, and a degree of homogeneity, in that all research participants were from the same professional group.[2]

The purpose of the interviews was not to explain, predict or generate theory, but to understand shared meanings by drawing from participants a picture of their experience of spirituality in relation to situations of loss, complete with the richness of detail and context that shaped their experience.[3] The interviews progressed alongside concurrent thematic analysis of meaningful patterns of these experiences illuminated in the texts of interview transcripts. Concurrent analysis helped determine sample size by reflecting sufficiency of overall transcript text in evidencing clarity and confidence that an adequate range of situations had been covered.[4]

The particularly focused nature of the study rendered it likely to support a small sample size.[5] Five interviews were conducted with nurses employed within a hospice, three with nurses employed in a nursing home and four with nurses employed in a community setting. Therefore in total 12 nurses were interviewed. Guest et al.[6] found that 12 interviews sufficed for most researchers who aim to discern themes concerning common views and experiences among a professionally homogenous group. Also, the sample heterogeneity in relation to practice settings was inclusive in its representation of all three sub-groups.[7] This contributed to adequacy in relation to the range of situations covered.[8]

CONDUCTING THE SEMI-STRUCTURED INTERVIEWS

In order to encourage dialogue to elicit participants' descriptions,[9] before commencing each interview I emphasized that the nature of the interview would be more like a conversation, rather than me asking a lot of questions. I also pointed out that I anticipated they would do most of the talking, because I was interested in their thoughts and experiences around the topics we were going to consider.

I tried to reduce the potential impact of the more 'professional' context of an interview rather than 'the everyday' nature of conversation[10] by using Field's[11] style of explaining to participants that there were no right or wrong answers and that they could share their thoughts and experiences as they perceived them, but that sometimes I would ask further questions to clarify or seek expansion on something they had mentioned.

Kahn[12] notes that, in traditional phenomenology, interviewers use a broad opening question that focuses on the phenomena under study. To this end a topic guide (see Table 4.1) was used to help direct conversation toward the subjects reflected in the study objectives, and so included spirituality, loss and personal resources. Guiding the direction of conversation in this way accounts for the 'semi-structured' nature of interview sessions. I found reflecting back my understanding of what participants had said, particularly from their earlier comments in the interview, was a useful source of clarification, both for me and for the participant, and a means of developing responses,[13] for example:

I think you implied…that your life experience has contributed to your understanding of spirituality…Has anything else contributed to your understanding of spirituality?

You've given…one example at least where you sensed the patient had a spiritual agenda…Are there other examples from practice…?

In order to conduct semi-structured interviews, arrangements were made to see each participant individually for a period of at least one hour. The interviews lasted between an hour and an hour and a half. Participants were all sent written information prior to consenting to interview, which explained that these events would be recorded on audiotape for later transcription. This provided a fuller record of the dialogue during the interview than written notes could provide. However, some notes were still taken during the interviews to record participants' non-verbal behaviour, and also to avoid interrupting the participant by noting issues mentioned that I was interested in following up. Audiotape recordings were independently transcribed. Transcripts were then audited against original audio tape recordings.[14]

In order to enable awareness of other factors that may impact responses at interview, participants were asked to complete a brief questionnaire to provide information regarding age, gender, professional qualifications, posts held since qualification as a registered nurse and any relevant post-registration training or education that they had undergone.

Table 4.1 Topic guide

Topic	Possible questions to initiate response	Potential prompts, clarification, development
Spirituality	What does the term spirituality mean to you?	…for herself/himself-within her/his working context
	How have you arrived at these understandings?	e.g. education, clinical assessment, experience, family values and beliefs
	What are your perceptions of spiritual need in practice?	e.g. evident, incidental, implicit, patient self sufficiency
	What experience have you had of spiritual care/support in practice?	…examples of these?
Loss	What do you understand by the term 'loss' in relation to your work?	e.g. inevitable, cumulative, related to death, related to disability
	What experience do you have of the issues that evolve in situations of loss?	e.g. despair, hope, perseverance, ultimate/existential question
	Give an example of a situation in which loss occurred	…how did you deal with this?
		…on reflection is there anything you would change now?
Personal resources	How do you deal with loss on a day-to-day basis?	e.g. therapeutic use of self, professional – more detached approach, referral
	What resources do you have personal access to as form(s) of support	e.g. professional support, personal resources
	Do you have a religious faith?	…which religion? practising?

ETHICAL CONSIDERATIONS IN COLLECTION AND STORAGE OF DATA

Research interviews involve human interaction that affects interviewees. Interviewing for research therefore has significant ethical and moral implications.[15] The inclusion of National Health Service staff as potential participants in the study meant that mandatory approval of the local Research Ethics Committee was sought prior to commencement of interviews. Written permission to access nurses employed in designated institutions and primary care trust was sought from appropriate managers. Nurses who were willing to participate in semi-structured interviews were provided with written information outlining the study. Written consent was gained from all participants and participation in interviews was voluntary. Interviews were conducted in an environment conducive to privacy, the site of which was negotiated with the participant and/or their manager. Participants had the right to withdraw from the interview if they so wished; however, no participant chose to do so. Sources of staff support were identified in case recollection related to accounts given at interview caused upset. Sources of support included clinical supervision or counselling. To ensure security of data, records that held the names of participants were kept separate from data that linked participants to codes. Research participants were reassured that the transcripts of interviews would not include any identifying features. In this way, in publishing details of data collected and my conclusions, the anonymity of participants is maintained.

RIGOUR

A researcher's self-conscious awareness of the values and experience they bring to their research contributes to rigour in that staying mindfully engaged in opening up research decisions and findings to public scrutiny reflects a transparency of process that promotes trustworthiness.[16] My account of the relevant knowledge and experience I brought to this study was presented in my account of fore-structure (see Chapter 3) and maintained in my research diary by my recording day-to-day thoughts and feelings generated, for example at interview encounters or on reading interview transcripts. Such information was helpful in providing insight into how situations were interpreted and made sense of.[17] Notes outlining my relationship with participants and any other influences that impacted research decisions helped maintain my awareness of personal subjectivity[18] in the interpretation of the meaning of these factors. These reflections and notes collectively constituted my research journal.

SUMMARY

In purposively inviting experienced nurses from practice environments that involve interface with situations of end of life care, a small sample size provided optimal-quality data, rich and thick enough to facilitate adequate understanding of the phenomenon studied. Emphasis on the conversational nature of interview, rather than having to respond to questions, allowed the participants to talk and thus share their thoughts and experiences around the topics being considered. Consideration and attention was given to both the ethical and moral implications of gaining and using information shared at interview and to the implications of my own values and experience on the research process. The process of data analysis is considered in depth in the following chapter.

REFERENCES

1. Cohen MZ. Introduction. In: Cohen MZ, Kahn DL and Steeves RH, editors. *Hermeneutic Phenomenological Research: a Practical Guide for Nurse Researchers*. Thousand Oaks, CA, London, New Delhi: Sage, 2000, 1–12.
2. Bryman A. How many qualitative interviews is enough? In: Baker SE and Edwards R, editors. *How Many Qualitative Interviews Is Enough? Expert Voices and Early Career Reflections on Sampling and Cases in Qualitative Research*. University of Southampton: National Centre for Research Methods Review Paper/Economic and Social Research Council, 2012 pp. 18–20.
3. Sorrell JM, Redmond GM. Interviews in qualitative nursing research: differing approaches for ethnographic and phenomenological studies. *Journal of Advanced Nursing*. 1995; **21**: 1117–22.
4. Benner P. The tradition and skill of interpretative phenomenology in studying health, illness, and caring practices. In: Benner P, editor. *Interpretive Phenomenology: Embodiment, Caring, and Ethics in Health and Illness*. Thousand Oaks, CA: Sage, 1994. pp, 99–127.
5. Bryman, op. cit.
6. Guest G, Bunce A and Johnson L. How many interviews are enough?: an experiment with data saturation and variability. *Field Methods*. 2006; **18**: 59–82.
7. Bryman, op. cit.
8. Benner, op. cit.
9. Jones SR and McEwen MK. A conceptual model of multiple dimensions of identity. In: Merriam SB *et al. Qualitative Research in Practice*. San Francisco, CA: Jossey-Bass, 2002, 163–74.
10. Kvale S and Brinkmann S. *Interviews: Learning the Craft of Qualitative Research Interviewing*. Thousand Oaks, CA: Sage, 2009.
11. Field D. *Nursing the Dying*. London: Routledge, 1989.
12. Kahn DL. (2000) How to conduct research. In: Cohen MZ, Kahn DL, Steeves RH, editors. *Hermeneutic Phenomenological Research: A Practical Guide for Nurse Researchers*. Thousand Oaks, CA: Sage, 2000, 57–70.
13. Kvale and Brickman, op. cit.
14. Tuckett A. Part II. Rigour in qualitative research: complexities and solutions [Interviewing]. *Nursing Researcher*. 2005; **13**(1): 29–42.
15. Kvale and Brickman, op. cit.
16. Finlay L. Through the looking glass: intersubjectivity and hermeneutic reflection. In: Finlay L and Gough B, editors. *Reflexivity: A Practical Guide for Researchers in Health and Social Sciences*. Oxford: Blackwell Science, 2003, 105–19.
17. Alaszewski A. *Using Diaries for Social Research*. London: Sage, 2006.
18. Jootun D, McGhee G and Marland GR. Reflexivity: promoting rigour in qualitative research. *Nursing Standard*. 2009; **23**(23): 42–6.

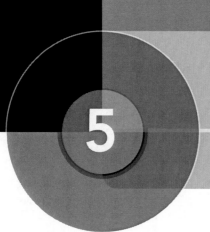

Analysis of experience shared

Clarke[1] refers to qualitative analysis as an intuitive, personal journey for the researcher in which meanings 'emerge' from the data as themes, and categories. Initial, informal analysis started at the point of conducting the interviews. Such a 'beginning of sorts' is inevitable in phenomenological studies, where interpretation of meaning begins on hearing the data at interview.[2] However, the dilemma of following a Heideggerian tradition of hermeneutic phenomenological research, is that the focus on the ontological study of 'Being', rather than knowledge production, results in a lack of specific method in approaching thematic analysis[3,4] (see Chapter 2). For this reason, a stepped approach, closely reflecting the scheme of Smith *et al.*,[5] was chosen as the means of methodically engaging with and interpreting data. This process of formal analysis is described below. My reflective diary and notes constituted a research journal, which provided an ordered account of my experience of making sense of research activities throughout the study.[6] Therefore, reflections that enrich the account of process of analysis are also included.

ANALYSIS OF TRANSCRIPTS OF INTERVIEW DATA

The intention of the analysis was to try to understand participants' experiences of spirituality as a resource for coping with loss. Reflective engagement with data, recorded in interview transcripts, enabled me to give an account of what I think the research participant is thinking, known as the double hermeneutic.[7] In this way, although findings aim to be accurate, they are somewhat tentative.[8] Repeated, or iterative, engagement with each transcript, allowing a shift from looking closely at a small piece of one text to seeing this in the context of the whole of that particular text and vice versa, demonstrates the process of the hermeneutic circle in guiding interpretation[9] (see Chapter 2). Similarly, individual texts are understood in relation to all texts, and vice versa.

STEP 1

The first step in formally commencing data analysis involved reading and re-reading the transcript. The audiotapes of all interviews were independently transcribed, and the accuracy of transcription was checked by listening to the appropriate audiotape while reading the transcript. Repeated listening to a recording triggered not only the recall of the voice of the participant, which was sustained during subsequent readings of the transcript, but also recall of the whole scenario of the interview ambience itself. Reliving the event in this way, together with repeatedly revisiting a transcript, allowed an increasing familiarity with the text, which Cohen *et al*.[10] describe as immersing oneself in the data.

STEP 2

The second step of analysis was one of initial noting. A wide margin was made on the right-hand side of each page of every transcript. Exploratory comments were noted in the margin during the readings of the transcript (see Table 5.1). Initially, these were descriptive in nature, identifying key words, phrases or explanations given by the participant that reflected their thoughts and experiences related to loss and spirituality. These comments embodied their experiences in relation to 'their world', and comprised thoughts not only on their current professional practice experience, but also, for many, additional comment on their past professional practice and/or their personal life experience.

Listening to audiotape recording of an interview while reading the transcript also provided the opportunity to note the manner of the participant's response against what was heard on the recording, such as laughter, sighs and thoughtful pauses. This enabled linguistic comment to be added (in italics) to exploratory comment, and initiated a focus on the way language was used by the participant (see Table 5.1). In looking closely at small pieces of text it was possible to see what Smith *et al*.[11] point out, that at times the way language is used and the content are clearly interrelated. An example was when research participant 10 was 'choked' when describing her emotional response to a card left by a patient. Metaphor could also be identified in this way, and provided a means of conveying strength of feeling or the scale of an experience. For example, when participant 2 described the impact of her son's suicide by saying, it 'threw my world just up in the air and it came crashing down in bits and pieces', she communicated some sense of the challenge that coping with this magnitude of loss presented. Most participants were inclined to be thoughtful in addressing the issues posed in their interview encounter. This was evident by pauses, before or in the throes of their response. Similarly, humour was used by all respondents at some time during their interview, often paradoxically when describing difficulty, or having difficulty in describing an experience.

Notes in my research diary also consider the impression of 'whole' interview style, and reflect that several participants varied in the way they used language. Such paralinguistic properties of speech are important in conveying either emotion or a nuance of meaning not evident in the text of transcripts. They also provide affirmation of the interpretation of meaning and emotion conveyed in the text,[12] such as the illustration above of participant 10 being 'choked'.

Research participant 2 was eloquent and confident in her responses, as was participant 4. They had both been registered nurses for many years, and so had a significant experience of practice. However, it was their comprehensive account of loss or illness suffered in their personal life which particularly conveyed their confidence in understanding what had shaped the development of their own spiritual growth and coping mechanisms.

Participants 7 and 11 were rather serious in their expression. Early in her interview participant 7 expressed the concern that 'I'm not explaining this very well', and participant 11 that she wasn't going to be 'very useful'. They appeared conscientious in wanting to 'get it right'.

Participants 3 and 8 tended to use humour more frequently than the group as a whole, although in different ways. Participant 3 used laughter almost too frequently, and on occasion finished with a sigh. This felt as if there was another agenda she was not sharing. Participant 8's use of humour was open in laughing at his recognition of paradox and contradiction.

Participant 12's demeanour and tone reflected her claim of 'I'm sort of struggling a bit' when it came to describing specific practice examples to illustrate general comments she had made.

Table 5.1 Exemplifying steps of analysis

Emergent themes	Transcript excerpt...	Exploratory comments
	Q: What do you think the term 'spirituality' means?	
	A: To me, it's a term that's often confused with religion, and although it can be about religious beliefs it's whatever gives that person, patient, their life meaning and purpose. So for some that might be religion and God, for some it might be digging the garden, for some it might be snowboarding! Anything that gives their life meaning and purpose, that's what it means to me.	confused with religion can be religious beliefs meaning and purpose religion/God digging garden snowboarding broad interpretation *smile*
Faith religious and non-religious		
	Q: I just wondered how you came to an understanding of the meaning of spirituality, in that way. How did you come to that?	
	A: Probably partly from academic courses and learning, partly from my own experience because I've worked in palliative care for about 15 years now, so a mixture of the two. And partly from practical experience of being with patients and families and seeing at the end of life what's important to them.	courses palliative care experience practical experience formal study with experience
	Q: Occasionally, somebody stands out in our mind – anything specific you can remember?	
	A: I do remember a lady who was a really, really devout Catholic for the whole of her life and while she was poorly, sort of took comfort from her religious beliefs and God, but when it got to about the last 5, 6 days of her life I don't think I've probably ever seen anybody more distressed because she was questioning everything – you know, if I've behaved in this way, led a good life, acted in this way, you know, I've led this good life, done everything right, never done anything wrong so why is this happening to me? And she was so distressed those last few days because she was questioning her belief, mainly in God, but in everything, you know – how she'd lived her life.	devout catholic *said with feeling* indication of degree of distress due to questioning doubt spiritual distress
Loss consequences for patients		

Her difficulty could be attributed to her being one of the youngest participants, and in that sense having less lived experience in practice to draw on. Participant 11, who was also a young respondent, had a similar struggle.

Following on from noting use of language, the transcript was revisited to add further comment, this time focused on trying to capture the research participant's overarching understanding of matters of loss and spirituality. These comments were added to those in the right-hand margin, but were underlined to differentiate them from descriptive notes of participant responses (see Table 5.1). Smith *et al.*[13] describe this activity as one of conceptual comment, requiring the researcher to be more interpretative and so begin to move away from explicit participant comment to conceptual annotating. Reflection produced tentative ideas or questions, and so opened up provisional meanings. There was a natural tendency for me to draw on my own experience and professional knowledge in framing these thoughts.

STEP 3

Step 3 involved the development of emergent themes. The data now constituted interview transcript text and exploratory comment or notes. This third stage required a shift to primarily dealing with the analysis of exploratory notes, rather than directly with transcript text. In this way, the quantity of detail was reduced, but the quality of complexity of data was maintained by the integral link between exploratory notes and transcript. Analysis was focused on a piece of text and related notes, rather than the 'whole' transcript, and so on 'parts' of data. These parts were ultimately reconfigured to form a new 'whole', as emergent themes were grouped later in the analysis. Themes are terms or phrases which succinctly embody the essence of the piece of transcript, and reflect both the participant's words and my interpretation of them.[14] Emerging themes were noted in the left-hand margin of the transcript alongside illustrative excerpts of text (see Table 5.1).

STEP 4

Searching for connections across emergent themes constituted step 4 of the process of analysis. Abstraction was the means of achieving this, and involved identifying patterns between emergent themes[15] so that they could be grouped into a smaller number of super-ordinate themes. Each super-ordinate theme was given a title that reflected the overarching focus of constituent themes.

STEP 5

Step 5 involved moving on to the next transcript. If new themes emerged as each transcript was analysed, these were recorded as before, or existing themes were strengthened by additional illustrative excerpts. Following the analysis of 12 interview transcripts, themes were not being further enriched by any new comment. Therefore, 12 interviews provided sufficiency of overall transcript text, and included an adequate range of situations across practice contexts.[16] Emergent themes were grouped into five super-ordinate themes (see Table 5.2).

Table 5.2 Super-ordinate and clustered themes

Super-ordinate theme	Themes emerging from data
Loss as a spectrum	Dominant issues of loss
	Consequences of loss for patients and their significant others
	Impact of loss on nurses
Belonging as the means of maintaining spiritual integrity	Accessing support for patient care
	Informal support for nurses
	Formal support for nurses
Belief as the pillar of spirituality	Meaning and purpose
	Religious and non-religious faith
	Faith as a resource to 'regulate distress'
	Personal philosophy as a coping strategy
Being a spiritual carer	Rapport and relationship as a spiritual resource
	Replenishment
Becoming proficient in spiritual care	Facilitation of religious practice as a spiritual resource
	Empowerment of patients
	Empowerment of support staff
	Personal loss; a source of enhanced understanding and positive growth

RESEARCH JOURNAL

Reflections relevant to the process and content of participant interviews are themed and are as follows:

CAUSE FOR THOUGHT

The interview process gave almost all participants cause for thought to the extent that they appeared thoughtful, or moved, or near tears at some point in the session. My response to these emotional moments varied. At times I found myself acknowledging my understanding of the difficulty of the situation they were describing, or that what they were saying was very moving, almost as an intuitive form of reassurance that it was alright for them to share such emotions in the interview. However, on other occasions, it felt more supportive for me to remain silent and leave space for them to accommodate how they felt. My appreciation for participants contributing to my research developed into a sense of privilege regarding what they were prepared to share with me. Most participants had shared something very personal that they had not shared, or would not normally share.

PARTICIPANTS' 'STORY'

My diary reflects a growing awareness of the pattern of each participant's account of their own spiritual development and how that impacts on their practice. There seemed to be a continuum of possibilities. Some arrived with a story to tell that reflected their own sense of a developed spirituality. Others began to voice an emerging story within the interview session, as if the opportunity to describe their understanding of spirituality in relation to loss exposed slithers of experience that suddenly shaped into a moment of spiritual insight and associated growth.

A couple had no real story to tell, but their interview experience seemed to have 'woken them up' to questions they had never considered and therefore not addressed as yet. The following examples illustrate my thoughts.

The fourth participant interviewed as if she came to tell her story. An undiagnosed illness in her early adult years, together with her evangelical religious views, drove the focus of a rather lengthy personal account. Her 'lived experience' of spirituality and loss seemed very powerful in her personal life because, although she did share some practice experience in relation to these phenomena, there seemed a continual return to her story of illness, religion and family. In some ways, participant 2 had a story to tell of an enduring Christian faith, a career centred round family needs and the loss of her son through suicide. This tapestry of personal experience had impacted her perspective on spirituality, and directly accounted for her choosing to work with end of life care patients. Participant 5's story is one of search, and openness in her approach to life and practice. I found her perceptive in understanding spirituality as timeless, spiritual awareness as heightened by situation, and philosophical in describing faith as understanding that all things happen for a reason.

On the other hand, participants 1 and 3 seemed to have a story that began to emerge within the interview session. In reflecting on the topics for discussion, they seemed to open up an awareness of their life experience that they had not realized before. For example, participant 1 vocalized for the first time what must have been kept as a tacit awareness, that when her first child was born she just knew there was a God. Participant 3 worked through the personal emotional challenges and achievements that she had with a particularly difficult patient and, in doing so, appeared to come to an understanding of her growth in a situation of sorrow.

Participants 11 and 12 were the youngest participants and each, in their own way, did not appear to have a story to tell 'yet'. When interviewing participant 11 I think I reverted to being an educationalist facilitating participation, rather than remaining purely in researcher mode, as she was finding the interview difficult and said, 'I don't think I'm going to be very useful.' She was in no way distressed, but seemed to be concerned that she would not be able to help. Facilitation 'worked' in getting started. Her comments reflected a nurse who practised holistic care and so implicitly addressed spiritual needs, but I do not think she had thought through spirituality as a concept integral to holistic philosophy herself. After interview she did say that the experience had 'caused her to think', and so, perhaps, had sown the 'seed of a story'. Participant 12 had attended a hospice palliative care course in which spirituality had constituted part of the content. She had therefore thought through terminology, and was able to give general comment on the topics for discussion. However, she had similar difficulty to participant 11 in exploring the application of these concepts in her practice. After the interview was finished, she said that the questions were difficult because 'you don't stop and think what you do and why you do it'. Once again such an insight might have seeded another 'story'.

SUMMARY

Interpretative analysis rests on the belief that human action is inherently meaningful. Empathetic identification with the participant helps generate an understanding of how their everyday 'lifeworld' is constituted. Similarly, their use of language is a key to understanding cultural norms. These forms of understanding contribute to interpreting the meanings of experience described by participants.

Participating in research interviews proved to be cathartic for some nurses, in that it enabled emotional response, and catalytic for others, in enhancing self-discovery by provoking thought.[17] Interpretative analysis of data has enhanced my own understanding of how nurses experience spirituality as a resource in coping with loss, details of which are addressed in Parts 2 and 3.

REFERENCES

1. Clarke B. Hermeneutic analysis: a qualitative decision trail. *International Journal of Nursing Studies.* 1999; **36**: 363–9.
2. Cohen MZ, Kahn DL and Steeves RH. How to analyze the data. In: Cohen MZ, Kahn DL and Steeves RH, editors. *Hermeneutical Phenomenological Research: a practical guide for nurse researchers.* London: Sage, 2000, 71–83.
3. Horrocks S. Hunting for Heidegger: questioning the sources in the Benner/Cash debate. *International Journal of Nursing Studies.* 2000; **37**(3): 237–43.
4. Rennie DL. Qualitative research: a matter of hermeneutics and the sociology of knowledge. In: Kopal M and Suzuki LA, editors. *Using Qualitative Research in Psychology.* London: Sage, 1999.
5. Smith JA, Flowers P and Larkin M. *Interpretative Phenomenological Analysis, Theory, Method and Research.* London: Sage, 2009.
6. Riessman CK. *Narrative Analysis.* Newbury Park, CA: Sage, 1993.
7. Brogden LM. Double Hermeneutic. In: Mills AJ, Durepos G and Wiebe E, editors. *Encyclopedia of Case Study Research.* Thousand Oaks, CA: Sage, 2010.
8. Kahn DL. Reducing bias. In: Cohen MZ, Kahn DL and Steeves RH. Editors. *Hermeneutic Phenomenological Research; a practical guide for nurse researchers.* Thousand Oaks, CA: Sage, 2000,: 85–92.
9. Cohen *et al.*, op. cit.
10. Ibid.
11. Smith *et al.*, op. cit.
12. Nygaard, LC and Lunders, ER. Resolution of lexical ambiguity by emotional tone of voice. *Memory and Cognition.* 2002; **30**(4), 583–93.
13. Smith *et al.*, op. cit.
14. Ibid.
15. Ibid.
16. Benner P. The tradition and skill of interpretative phenomenology in studying health, illness, and caring practices. In: Benner P, editor. *Interpretive Phenomenology: Embodiment, Caring, and Ethics in Health and Illness.* Thousand Oaks, CA: Sage, 1994, 99–127.
17. Heron J. *Six Category Intervention Analysis.* 3rd ed. Guildford: University of Surrey, 1989.

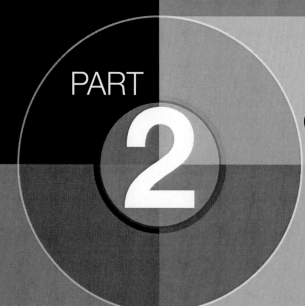

PART 2

IMPACT OF LOSS AS A CONTEXT OF CARE

Every time there's a change or transition in life there are many losses involved…but obviously there are spectrums of loss… (participant 8)

Nurses participating in the study were encouraged to share their understanding of loss and to give examples of experiences that had shaped that understanding. It was evident from their descriptions that caring for people with chronic and terminal illness was an experience infused with issues of loss. One nurse suggested there are spectrums of loss, and so implied the relevance of significance in relation to what is being, or has been, lost. This highlights the importance of understanding loss from the patient's perspective; for example, a small incremental loss sometimes triggers what may seem a disproportionate emotional response in a patient if it signifies decline.

There were a number of similarities in the impact of loss in all three practice environments. First, the consequences of loss for patients were similar. Second, nurses from each of the different practice settings gave examples of situations where additional support was needed for patients to help them cope with loss. This support was arranged or facilitated by the nurses rather than provided by them. Yet another similarity was that of the emotional impact on nurses of repeated exposure to situations of loss.

However, there were also some differences identified between practice environments. In particular they differed in dominant issues of loss, which in turn influenced the dynamics of the teams in which nurses belonged and looked to for support.

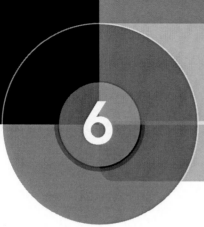

Consequences of loss for patients and their significant others

6

Nurses' experiences of end of life care indicated that the consequences of loss for their patients were similar, regardless of the environment they practised in. Descriptions reflect the enduring physical, psychological, social and spiritual effects of loss that have to be coped with. Significant loss is described as a process of change, not only for the person themselves, but also for their significant others:

Well it's a change in your life, isn't it, so whether it's a chronic illness or an actual loss, it's a complete change to your life and the people around you, their lives as well, because you know generally speaking people have got friends or family who…and they work as a little network and if something happens to one of them it affects everybody (participant 12)

Loss is often incremental in nature, particularly in those with advanced chronic disease. Incremental loss is driven by, and evidence of, deterioration:

I've a lady with MS…her mind is perfect, she can still work and does computer work and things like that but the fact that she can't empty her catheter bag for herself any more, or… it's those little bits of your life [that] are just slowly being taken away, it's like a constant loss but over a long period of time…picking up a cup for example…she used to be able to do that 3 weeks ago, but can't do that today… (participant 12)

…if their condition deteriorates further so that one day…someone has been able to feed themselves and the next day they can't, (participant 5)

SOCIAL DEATH

Currer[1] describes social death as an aspect of a relationship, and of how one person perceives another. It is seen as the culmination of a sequence of events that results in an individual no longer actively participating in others' lives.[2] Nurses' descriptions indicating the consequences of loss for patients illustrate a variety of such sequences, for example, apart from observing the physical deterioration of patients, the following respondent describes how the dying patient becomes more introspective and socially isolated, even from those closest to them:

> ...I think there is a very big change in the person physically, either extreme weight loss or extreme weight gain through being on steroids. People losing their hair, physical things, and also, I think when people are terminally ill they don't tend to be interested any more in everyday things and they're obviously very much occupied by their impending death... so they don't want to talk about things that they perhaps used to talk about with a partner or friend (participant 1)

The slow dissolution of personhood through terminal illness[3] is implied in the following description of how family members face the loss of the person they knew, prior to biological death. It is also another example of the countenance of social death:

> ...when somebody is terminally ill and they are obviously totally different people than they were before and everything is changed...people say to you 'he is no longer my husband', 'she is no longer my wife, she is just...a completely different person'...I suppose that is loss already before the actual death (participant 1)

In situations where patients have dementia, cognitive decline precedes physical decline. Therefore friends and relatives endure the loss of the relationship they had with the person for a potentially lengthy period before physical decline ultimately results in death. In this way, social death is a situation relatives live with, rather than encounter for the first time as biological death draws near:

> ...[the] family of these people are suffering loss, particularly somebody who's got dementia, because the person they knew they're losing even though they are still there, it's not the same person, and learning to cope with that loss can be quite hard... (participant 10)

ANTICIPATORY GRIEF

Incremental physical changes, together with social isolation, exemplify the cumulative loss that occurs through the palliative phase of living with dying, and the final decline that terminates in death. The process of dealing with these losses is described as a transition in which all those involved somehow undergo a preparation, a gradual coming to terms with and accepting the inevitability of losses associated with their own, or their relative's, situation. One nurse describes how professional carers contribute to this preparation, which is particularly important for those who will be 'left behind' following the death. This period of transition is about dealing with, and hence coping with, loss. Paradoxically, in this process relationships are seen to undergo a preparation for a loss, which is primarily the loss of those relationships. This paradox has been described by some theorists[4] as anticipatory grief:

> I think there's an adjustment that goes on, certainly in the community, when you're caring for what starts as palliative care, if you like, we're coming to the palliative care stage and then we move onto the terminal care stage. And I think during that time, if you're looking at spouses or carers or family, children, in some ways there's a preparation that goes on for that loss, with the carers, with those that are left behind. There's that preparation. When death is known, and you're involved with that as a professional, I think there is…you can see a transition going on and I know Kubler-Ross talks about this acceptance thing, but I think it doesn't come at the end…, I think this comes very much when palliative care starts and I think the individual, if you like, is already coping with that loss, is already beginning to deal with that loss. So I don't think it happens at death at all, that's not the cut-off point, that's not the loss,…they've begun to lose that partnership, that companionship, that decision-making, that…that's happening, that's a gradual thing that's happening (participant 9)

LOSS OF CONTROL

Deterioration results in patients needing more support. An increasing dependence on others culminates in a sense of loss of control. The sense of frustration felt by patients who can no longer do what they could is evident in the following description:

> …there's loss of independence, loss of the ability to function as they were previously functioning. I guess a lot of elderly people have talked about the frustration of loss, not being able to do what they could do and finding it very hard, even though mentally they're…they feel like a 20-year-old but their body isn't and they hate that. So in that sense that's obviously a big loss, not being able to do things…you feel like you can, but obviously your body can't (participant 11)

As the need for support increases, the roles held by the patient are usually gradually relinquished.[5] However, personality theory suggests that individuals tend to either have an internal locus of control and feel they are largely in control of their lives, or have an external focus and attribute control to some other agent, such as God, or other people.[6] Evidence suggests that where people have had an internal locus of control this tendency is likely to increase until middle age.[7]

A hospice nurse describes a scenario in which a patient who had not only been in charge of his own life but had controlled those of his wives and families, strongly resisted relinquishing his controlling status, to the point of becoming aggressive. The pathology of his condition meant that at times he was lucid and others not, and the nurse describes how, regardless, he agitated for control. This man's 'fight' to remain in charge may reflect his need to be himself, to live with dying as he has lived his life. Nurses can be uncomfortable with these situations. They tend to associate a 'good death' with being 'at peace' rather than struggle.[8] However, even Kubler-Ross,[9] who included 'acceptance' as the final stage of her theory of living with dying, did not specify that this would be done 'quietly':

We've had a gentleman…with a brain tumour and a fairly young family, who – I think he'd been quite a controlling person – and I think was still trying to run his family while he was here and wanted to leave on occasions. That was quite difficult I think because some of the time he was well aware of what was going on and other times he really wasn't, there was still this agitation with him all the time, he knew he had sort of lost his role in the family really and he couldn't be there with them, he couldn't be keeping his eye on what was going on and he couldn't organize them all, and that was quite difficult for his wife because occasionally he was quite aggressive with it as well. Which was quite difficult in a way I think for the children and his wife, really quite frightening obviously for them. And that…he had a wife, he had an ex-wife, and I think children with them and they were all coming in to visit…and he was still trying to run everything just as he liked…and it was difficult all round with all the family members and trying to help them, and trying to help him really, to understand that he wasn't well enough to just go and carry on as normal (participant 7)

Anger as an emotional response to helplessness is most effectively dealt with if the nurse remains calm.[10] Information is used to facilitate coping by allowing preparation for inevitable loss, and post bereavement visiting as a means of promoting coping by assuaging any sense of abandonment, for example:

We understand that in certain situations people feel quite angry because they're helpless. Loss has occurred or is going to occur and there's nothing they can do about it, so they take their frustrations out in anger. But you get to know these people and afterwards they'll apologise if they've been angry towards you, but you just know it's a part of the process and you just have to help them through it really, and explain and remain calm. And I think with the terminal patient if you explain everything, what's going to happen, I think that helps them come to terms with the loss, preparing them for it. It doesn't make it easier, but I think it just makes it easier to cope, understanding helps to prepare people for it. Doesn't mean to say they're going to like it! – But I think with a little bit more understanding. And we try…if possible, we can't always do it, but if we have been looking after somebody palliatively and they die, we try and go back to see the relatives a few weeks afterwards to see how they are. Just so they know that we used to come in every day and see you but we are still around, we haven't just abandoned you because your loved one has died. I think that can be quite beneficial to people coping with loss (participant 10)

CULTURE AND CONSEQUENCES OF LOSS

Roman Catholicism is a particularly strict form of Christian culture. Spiritual distress as a consequence of loss of religious faith by a devout Catholic patient seemed really harrowing. The respondent, a very experienced nurse, implied that she had never experienced nursing anyone as distressed before:

> I do remember a lady who was a really, really devout Catholic for the whole of her life and while she was poorly sort of took comfort from her religious beliefs and God, but when it got to about the last 5/6 days of her life I don't think I've probably ever seen anyone more distressed because she was questioning everything – you know, if I've behaved in this way, led a good life, acted in this way, you know I've led this good life, done everything right, never done anything wrong, so why is this happening to me? And she was so distressed those last few days because she was questioning her belief, mainly in God, but in everything, you know, how she'd lived her life (participant 6)

The Catholic Church places major emphasis on the sacraments and the symbolic significance of worship. This life is considered merely a beginning, with death providing the conduit to 'fullness of life'.[11] The sacrament of extreme unction performed by a priest for a dying Catholic symbolizes forgiveness, healing and reconciliation. However, this patient seemed no less distressed after her priest's visits.

> …I mean I've seen people over the years who have been distressed and have been able to seek comfort, but I think she sticks in my mind because she died distressed, she was so distressed (participant 6)

Evidence suggests that there are cultural differences in patterns of coping with loss, even in societies that share fundamentally the same religious base.[12] Similarly, Walter[13] outlines the differences that occur within a single culture of 'Englishness'. One participant exemplifies cultural difference in comparing the rather melodramatic style of grief, which he observed when previously working in South America, with the spectrum of English cultural response to loss that he has experienced in his current practice environment:

> Well I worked in South America…and out there when someone dies it's literally wailing, people collapsing on the floor fainting and incredibly melodramatic and everyone knows, the whole street will know about it and everyone comes and visits and they all cry and everyone's there, and it's just the end of the world, seriously big time! People throwing themselves in the grave and all that sort of stuff, it is pretty amazing. And so I've seen that. And having the wake, people have a wake and everyone from far afield comes and has to pay their respects and that sort of stuff. So that's one extreme, and then the other extreme is where you see people in this country who…it's done and dusted, and they have to go on and get themselves busy sorting out what do we do now, this kind of no emotion shown

and they have to get on with their lives and they have to get on with tasks of sorting out what's the next thing to be done. So there are extremes of reaction to loss. And that's not to say that either one or the other is right or wrong, it's just the way cultures and societies and personalities have formed that person to react in that way...but even within English culture you've got a spectrum of response to it [loss] (participant 8)

SUMMARY

Consequences of loss for patients were similar, regardless of practice context. As well as physical deterioration driving incremental loss, the psychological challenges of loss included anger, loss of control and the paradox of anticipatory grief for patients and their significant others. Social death provides a potentially lengthy challenge for relatives, and loss of faith as a coping strategy can result in severe spiritual distress in a patient. Culture impacts patterns of coping with loss, and varies across the subcultures that constitute 'Englishness'.

REFERENCES

1. Currer C. *Responding to Grief, Dying, Bereavement and Social Care*. Basingstoke: Palgrave, 2001.
2. Mulkay M and Ernst J. The changing profile of social death. *European Journal of Sociology*. 1991; **32**: 172–96.
3. Habgood J. *Being a Person: Where Faith and Science Meet*. London: Hodder & Stoughton, 1998.
4. Rando TA. Living and learning the reality of a loved one's dying: traumatic stress and cognitive processing in anticipatory grief. In: Doka K and Davidson J, editors. *Living with Grief When Illness Is Prolonged*. Bristol: Taylor Francis, 1997, 33–50.
5. Lugton J. Support processes. In: Lugton J and Kindlen M, editors. *Palliative Care: The Nursing Role*. Edinburgh: Churchill Livingstone, 1999, 89–113.
6. Rotter JB. Internal versus external control of reinforcement: a case history of a variable. *American Psychologist*. 1990; **45**(4): 489–93.
7. Schultz DP and Schultz SE. *Theories of Personality*. Belmont, CA: Wadsworth Thomson, 2005.
8. McNamara B, Waddell C and Colvin M. The institutionalization of the good death. *Social Science and Medicine*. 1994; **39**: 1501–8.
9. Kubler-Ross E. *On Death and Dying*. London: Tavistock, 1970.
10. Sheldon F. *Psychosocial Palliative Care*. Cheltenham: Stanley Thornes, 1997.
11. Green J. *Death with Dignity Volume II*. London: Macmillan, 1993.
12. Wikan U. Bereavement and loss in two Muslim communities: Egypt and Bali compared. *Social Science and Medicine*. 1988; **27**(5): 451–60.
13. Walter T. *On Bereavement: the Culture of Grief*. Buckingham: Open University Press, 1999.

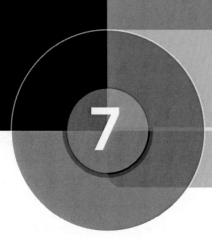

Accessing support to help patients cope

...so you have to think about...who can help (participant 11)

Interview accounts included a number of examples of situations from all three practice environments, in which patients needed additional support that was arranged, or facilitated, by the nurses rather than provided by them. When this occurred nurses looked to other professional colleagues from the wider interprofessional team, or additional support from relatives to help patients access the care they needed. Interprofessional working is promoted in situations where two or more professionals from different disciplines improve the quality of patient care through better collaboration.[1] Patients are central to such collaborative practice, as are their significant others.[2]

ARRANGED SUPPORT

One respondent from the hospice described the sort of situation that would generally warrant nurses referring a patient for counsellor support. However, she also indicates the value of pastoral support from the Chaplain:

I think sometimes, perhaps, people sort of coming to terms with or wanting to talk about their impending death...if we feel – sorry I'm now sort of talking about 'we' as nursing staff in general in the hospice – often refer to the family support team, which may consist of counsellors. Although, I personally, even if it's non-religious, I myself would probably speak to the Chaplain first of all because he's also very good in non-religious spiritual care (participant 1)

There were a number of examples of situations where nurses needed support from others to help them with patients who are mentally ill. The first example, given by a respondent practising in the nursing home, was where the challenge for staff was helping a patient who had schizophrenia to stay calm. They were resourceful in finding a volunteer from a local church to spend time with her. As the patient was religious this form of companionship would have provided familiarity and the comfort of an additional person to talk to. They also sought professional support in arranging for a Community Psychiatric Nurse to visit regularly to help staff manage the patient's particular mental health needs within what was a general practice environment:

> I remember a woman who…it was quite difficult…she had schizophrenia and she was here because she also had physical diseases as well. And she needed someone to talk to a lot of the time to keep her calm to stop her from going where they shouldn't do and that sort of thing. And hence, because the carers found her quite difficult to manage, the trained nurses were spending a lot of their time with her and so, because like we were spending so much time with her it was taking time away from other people who needed us. And the nurses could see there was a need to try and get outside support for her. She was a religious lady, we ended up being able to get her a volunteer from the local church who used to come and visit. And then we also got a CPN to come and visit her…regularly as well. And even though it was still quite difficult to manage her within the home in the time constraints we had made it easier and she was more calmer (participant 3)

A second patient scenario, described by the same nurse as not being as 'drastic', still indicates the additional time needed to support patients who are mentally ill. This patient was depressed and although her week was interspersed with visits and social activities from outside the nursing home, the patient's mood was very low in those periods when she was not being visited. The nurse's account also indicates how difficult it is to encourage hope, when a patient's memory is unreliable and limits their ability to 'look forward':

> …and I think of a lady who's still with us, and I mean she is very low in mood a lot of the time…you go in to see her to do what you need to do and she'll sort of say something like she needs help from carers to do this, that and the other, but she doesn't want to press her buzzer because she's being a nuisance. And I don't know, she……she's obviously depressed, she's on antidepressants which haven't made that much of a difference…she's got a visitor who takes her to the hospice service once a week, and she has a daughter-in-law – her family don't see her because they can't cope with her being in a nursing home… her daughter-in-law visits a couple of times a week. She works full time and so she can't really manage to do any more, and then she [the patient] has a friend who visits once a fortnight. I mean it's all so difficult for her, with this disease she's got, her memory isn't very good so its difficult to try and orientate her to look forward. You come in the morning and it's 'oh, what's going on today'. She'll say what day it is, sometimes it'll be right, sometimes it won't. It's very difficult because even if, like, she's got a week where she's doing something, social activities or visitors every day, she'll still have a morning where she's really low because nobody comes to visit her… (participant 3)

The support networks available for patients in community and their benefits are outlined by one participant, but she goes on to describe how personal belief may provide an inherent source of support for patients who are philosophical in understanding death as a natural progression of living:

There's definitely support networks from our palliative care team, you know, Macmillan nurses and other alternative kind of therapies and things, I think there's lots of support goes on there, meeting people with, you know, similar diagnosis, prognosis, that all… they're all things that people draw on for support, not…I could say not spiritual, I didn't mean not spirituality, but I was going to say…all some people need maybe is their spirituality, their belief in this is life, this is the natural progression, however I die, I'm meant to die at the end of the day and they maybe don't…I don't know, maybe they don't have that adjustment to acceptance because it's already inherent in them if you know what I mean? People say no, it's got to happen and however it happens it's not the actual happening, it's maybe the process (participant 9)

Sheldon[3] outlines a number of factors around the time of death that are associated with a poor outcome of bereavement for relatives and significant others. These include multiple bereavements and untimely/unexpectedly early deaths. Consequently support that spans the event of death is considered beneficial for the bereaved.[4] This was exemplified in a scenario in which a 39-year-old man suffering from multiple sclerosis was admitted to the nursing home to die. His mother was distraught, given that his impending death heralded the loss of a second adult child. Additional nursing services for the terminal phase of her son's life also provided increased support for the mother. A responsive GP and advice from Macmillan services enhanced support further:

We had a young man die here…he was thirty-nine and his mum really needed a lot of support, it was the second child she was about to lose…they let us have two trained nurses on the floor while he was terminally ill for a few days. So you've got more people to support his mum, to go in there, so somebody was always with her. We have used the Macmillan nurses from the hospice for advice, although we're quite confident in defining our own care to be honest. But the resource is there. The GP, our GP at the time, was very good, he'd come in daily (participant 5)

Following her son's death additional resources were used to enhance her last memory of her son, and for her support in bereavement:

We had an aromatherapist working here then who came in after he'd passed away and laid him out all very nicely and made the room look very nice, so we were able to do that for her (his mother). And we organized support for her afterwards through the Macmillan nurses as well (participant 5)

Nurses also arranged visits for nursing home residents if it helped them come to terms with their situations of loss, for example, they arranged for a resident to visit the bungalow she had lost when she moved into the nursing home. This helped her come to terms with it no longer belonging to her:

We had a lady that was very upset about losing her bungalow. And in the end, through the care manager…she actually went back to see this bungalow, they had her outside the bungalow and she realized it was no longer hers. It was very hard, upsetting work (participant 5)

FACILITATION AS SUPPORT

Additional beneficial support was also provided at the time of bereavement in a community scenario. Here the community nurse was the 'go-between' for the bereaved family and the funeral director, and so facilitated the family's need for more time with their deceased mother. The funeral director also agreed to accommodate the family's unusual request to collect their mother's body at night. In negotiating these arrangements the family was allowed to cope with their loss in their own way. Her actions were perceived as sensitive support by the family:

They were at a complete loss as to what happened next…I do remember having to say to them we need a funeral director and we need to phone and…etc etc…And was telling them all about this funeral director and things and they were taking it all on board, but they then pushed it all back at me: 'Could you do it, we can't do it.' And I remember thinking these are mature women and a mature husband, intelligent people, but they couldn't pick up the phone, so I remember ringing…and then sort of having this three-way phone conversation with the funeral director and the family…And they clearly did not want that body removed. And they said yes, they realized it had to happen but they hadn't had long enough…they did know how to deal with their loss but not in the way that, if you like, as a professional I needed it to be dealt with…Because I'd always thought…although I'd never put a time frame on it, but I thought perhaps these days people want the job done…I don't know. It was really quite bizarre…we did agree on a time, they ordered the body to be removed at night as well, not during daytime hours…I don't know why, I didn't really explore that (participant 9)

The nurse went on to explain how this event, which she had found bizarre at the time and which was one that she had not really understood, had been a lesson for her in raising awareness of how she had assumed relatives would take similar action to cope with bereavement when in fact, facilitating their individual coping strategies was the most effective form of support:

But I have to say I did get home late, probably about two hours, but I remember going home thinking that was quite a good job done really…I had the [most] wonderful memorable letter of thanks that I've ever received in the whole of my nursing career…from that family in that they used words like 'sensitive' and 'calmness' and I just thought, well… that was a bit of a learning curve for me too…and I keep it on me…because it was just…it pulled me up, I think. Because I obviously had some assumptions, didn't I, you know, once death occurs the body is removed and people kind of get on with it, but they needed to get on with it their way…Even though I kind of couldn't understand it at the time, but isn't that what it's about, you know, we're all individuals aren't we and you know people if that's what they want, then if it's humanly possible then that's hopefully what they get, because [death] it's quite an event (participant 9)

FAMILY RESOURCED SUPPORT

Family relationships played a significant role in supporting patients in a number of respondents' accounts. One respondent employed in a nursing home describes using the supportive relationships within families who are 'onside' as a strategy to help clients cope with their situation:

And if you've got family that's what I call 'onside' then you use them, you know, don't abuse them but you actually use that relationship to help the client to cope with the situation (participant 4)

More specifically, three scenarios, all given by hospice nurses, described how a particular member of the patient's family was able to help them deal with unfinished business. In the first instance, staff, intuitively aware that a patient was troubled, spoke to her family and eventually managed to elicit details of estrangement between the patient and her brother. When asked, the patient was keen to see her brother. The brother agreed to visit and so appeased his sister's need for reconciliation before she died:

And we just felt there was something troubling her that we hadn't recognized…And we spoke to her family about it…they eventually said there is someone that mum hasn't seen for many years, and they told us about the brother and that they'd parted on bad terms, and the family didn't feel that they could talk to her about it. So we said is it alright if we talk to her about it, so they agreed…I…had some time with her on my own and I broached the subject, and she just started crying, and I just let her cry. And I said, would you like us to try and contact your brother and she said, 'oh yes please'. And the relief in her voice was just – just said it all…we contacted the brother and he came in and it was a very emotional reunion and she died the next day…in peace (participant 2)

A second example was described by a nurse who noticed a marked change in the mood of a patient in his care. The nurse persevered in investigating the cause and found that the patient wanted to see his daughter as a matter of urgency. The patient's meeting with his daughter was lengthy, and upsetting for both of them, but afterwards he was no longer troubled. When this patient died his daughter voiced her appreciation of the nurse's facilitation of the conversation that addressed what was clearly a significant issue for them both, and one of spiritual distress for the patient:

…there was a gentleman who I remember one morning, normally quite a jolly and happy-go-lucky chap, but this morning he just seemed really down and quiet…I would say possibly even tormented by something…We went through everything and there were no symptoms that could account for…the way he was looking. And so I said, is there something on your mind? And he didn't say anything, he just kept quiet, which obviously meant that there was something on his mind. And I said, I'm happy to hear what you say, you don't have to say anything, but I'm quite happy to just talk to you about it. And he said, I need to see my daughter, and I said, 'OK, would you like me to contact your daughter' and he said, 'yes I want to see her today, it's really important'…so I phoned his daughter and said he's a little bit down and he wants to see you, it's quite important, so that afternoon she came. He was in a side room so I took her in there and they had about one and a half hours together. And eventually she came out…obviously in tears… and he'd obviously been in tears and been really upset, but the torment was gone…And when he died…she thanked me for calling her in, she didn't say what it was about or anything, but it was a very significant conversation they'd had and she felt I was able to facilitate that. So I thought that, for me, was a patient in spiritual distress at that point and by doing something very simple – all I could do was just arrange something to happen (participant 8)

The third example differed in that the patient, who was very agitated and described by the nurse as actively dying, was not reticent about his need, which was to visit his home because there were things he needed to do. He was also very specific in who he wanted to go with. They were a supportive family and the nurse arranged the visit as he requested. The impact was a marked change in that he returned to die in a much more relaxed frame of mind:

We had a gentleman once who was clearly very, very unwell and…actively dying, who was absolutely adamant he was going home one morning, not to stay at home, just for a visit home because there were things he needed to do. So we talked to him about it and phoned the two daughters and two sons-in-law…and said, your dad wants to, he's absolutely adamant, he's getting himself out of bed and getting ready to go and he really needs to. So they said, oh well we will organize it, come over to fetch him and bring him home. But he wanted to go home with one of the son-in-laws and not the daughters, whatever it was he wanted to do at home it was really important to him…he wanted a man to go and deal with it with him, and I think to be honest he went home to put some affairs in order, because he came back and was a different person, completely settled, and the daughters even said it, that whatever it was he'd needed to do, it completely settled him. So he went from being quite agitated mentally to coming back and being completely relaxed, which the family appreciated as well (participant 7)

SUMMARY

A number of nurses' experiences implied a limit, or boundary, to the means of fulfilling patient need. Family relationships played a significant role in supporting patients, particularly where members of a patient's family helped them deal with unfinished business. The many facets of holistic end of life care inevitably mean that no one professional group can address all aspects of care. Recognition of personal and professional boundaries, together with referral to others, was in itself spiritual care directed towards meeting patients' needs in coping with loss.

REFERENCES

1. Barr H. *Interprofessional Education Today, Yesterday and Tomorrow*. London: Occasional Paper 1 Learning and Teaching Support Network for Health Sciences and Practice, 2002.
2. Cox K and James V. Professional boundaries in professional care. In: Payne S, Seymour J and Ingleton C, editors. *Palliative Care Nursing: Principles and Evidence for Practice*. Berkshire: McGraw Hill/Open University Press, 2008, 554–72.
3. Sheldon F. Bereavement. In: Fallon M and O'Neill B, editors. *ABC of Palliative Care*. London: British Medical Journal, 1998, 63–5.
4. Currer C. Care at the end of life and in bereavement. In: Adams R, Dominelli L and Payne M, editors. *Critical Practice in Social Work*. 2nd ed. Basingstoke: Palgrave Macmillan, 2009, 368–78

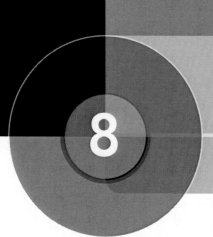

Impact of loss on nurses

8

The impact of loss on participants was evident in their responses, and affirms current knowledge in relation to the emotional challenge that such situations evoke,[1] as well as the culture of stress and coping in end of life care contexts.[2] When speaking of loss from their own perspective, nurses were referring to the death of a patient or person they knew.

GRIEF AS A CONSEQUENCE OF CARING ABOUT PATIENTS

Bobinac *et al.*[3] differentiate between the concepts of caring for another person and caring about them. Caring for a person is present in people providing care, and caring about them is present in the larger group of people who have a social relationship with the person who is ill, whether or not they provide care. A community nurse describes, in general terms, how in getting to know their patients over a period of time, the relationship between nurse and patient that develops takes on a duality, one of a professional carer who is also a sort of 'friend'. Campbell[4] describes this relationship as one of 'moderated love' that reflects consistent, skilled and informed concern. Where 'moderated love' constitutes caring for another over a lengthy duration, 'companionship' may include the nurse in the larger group who has a social relationship with a patient. In this way, a nurse could be described as caring for and caring about their patient. The death of a patient is therefore a situation of loss for the nurse as well as the family, but as the professional it is for the nurse to support relatives in their loss.

Well loss…if you know somebody and they pass away then it does affect the people who are looking after them, it affects the family, and as a nurse we kind of have to support the family by doing bereavement visits and that sort of thing, you know, to help to deal with their loss and prepare them for a future possibly on their own, but to know that they've got the support of us as well. But obviously as a team it does…you, know, when you have looked after somebody for so long they've become almost…although they are a patient, they've become like a friend at the same time and if somebody dies it does affect you. It can be very upsetting and sort of difficult but at the same time we have to be professional and step in and help with the family…husbands, wives, children…to support them (participant 12)

More specific reference to the challenge of loss for a nurse who befriends a patient was described by a respondent employed within the nursing home. She seemed to be comparing the length of time she had known the patients before they died with the length of time she had worked at the nursing home, hence implying the long duration of these relationships. Grief is a reflection of the attachments formed between people.[5] This is exemplified in the pain suffered as a cost of investment by this nurse in close relationships with patients who later died. This is very personal to the nurse as she uses 'I' when speaking of her loss. She explains, in referring to the death of her mother, how the impact of loss at work is compounded by the suffering of loss in one's personal life at the same time. Despite the investment of herself in care, again the nurse is very clear about professional boundaries. Although, initially comparing close relationships with patients to being like family, she then goes on to affirm that she is aware of the difference. The problem of closeness and distance wherever care is professional is seen by Campbell[6] as particularly difficult in nursing. The nurse is perhaps affirming this difficulty when she describes how although she does not have close bonds with all patients, she looks after all patients professionally:

…one that I lost a little while ago, he was here the whole time I've been here, and I've been here 11 years, and he 10 years. Daphne died this year and she was here 8 years… and…you're building relationships and each time they go that is a loss. And particularly if you've got loss going on in your own life, that's another thing. My mother died this year, it was difficult. We had a couple of ladies…died at the same time, and my mum was in South Africa and I can remember one day having this bizarre phone call with my sister in Johannesburg and the doctor hadn't turned in, [and the sister said] oh we'll wait and see what happens tomorrow, and I just lost it…so it is painful when they die. Yes, they're like family but they're not family. It's that…there is a divide, of course, and there are one or two that I've got bits of them around my home, you know, little trinkets that they've given me over the years…you know, Christmas they give you bits…you don't bond with all of them, you know, you do your best, you put your professional hat on and you look after all of them professionally but there are the odd one or two that really get under your skin, and you think they could have been friends if we'd met in a different era or sphere or something (participant 4)

Similarly, the implication of nurses finding death particularly hard if they connect with the patient in a personal way is exemplified by a community nurse. In this case the patient was also a nurse, and in relating to the patient as 'one of us' the personal association with a member of the same profession may have made the death particularly upsetting for the respondent. Although she had looked after dying patients before, this was the first time she was the 'lead' nurse for a dying patient and in that sense, this situation was 'special'. Staff sickness in an already small team had further intensified this nurse's engagement with the patient during her terminal phase of care. The respondent was middle aged and her patient, who was an experienced nurse, may well have been of a similar age. The bond that had developed between patient and nurse is evident in that, first, the patient took the trouble to write a card of appreciation to be given to the respondent after her death, and second, the degree of emotion that this card generated in the nurse when she read it. Davies and Oberle's[7] study found that preservation of the nurse's own integrity was central to her being able to care for patients living with dying at home. Sharing frustrations with colleagues was one means of achieving this. Therefore, the nurse's intense sense of loss in this case may have been assuaged had working circumstances been normal, and so, provided opportunity for more support in both sharing the emotional burden of terminal care, and some respite in the intensity of attending to this patient:

…I'd spent such a long time with her and I found it quite hard when she died and quite upsetting. But I wasn't expecting the card (of thanks from the deceased patient) I think that came probably as a bit of a shock to me which probably added to my sense of loss with her. I don't know whether it was because she was a fellow nurse as well, 'one of us'. But perhaps because I'd just spent so much time with her in the few weeks leading up to her death (participant 10)

MANAGING EMOTIONAL UPHEAVAL

The description of this particular situation also exemplifies how, apart from an initial release of emotion following the death of a patient, later events can trigger emotional upheaval. Privacy in coping with tears as a response to grief is apparent in the nurse's relief that she didn't open the card in the house and break down in front of the patient's husband:

…her husband left a message for us to go around and see him and I went round to see him and he gave me a card from her that she had written before she died, thanking me for her care. And for everything that we'd done, and I'm glad I didn't open it in the house, I took it away and opened it, I drove the car around the corner and sat and opened it and it just made me burst into tears, it was just too much, really. Because she was prepared for losing her life and she tried her utmost to prepare everybody else (participant 10)

A number of other nurses gave examples of how once out of sight of patients and relatives their professional ethos gives way to the emotional expression of grief. They were quite choked with emotion as they gave their accounts of these incidents. Walter[8] describes contemporary private grief among those of white English culture as that in which the pain of grief is expressed out of the public eye, and that getting on with life is the way in which individuals distract themselves from grief in public. He further explains that Stroebe and Schut's[9] dual process model of coping with bereavement describes how individuals oscillate between expressing their grief in private and carrying on as normal in public. The nurse's comment above, and the following quotations from respondents, all of whom Walter would categorize as of white English culture, describe moments of private grief. One community nurse describes how she stopped her car so that she could weep:

I had a great rapport with this family and was actually there when she died and I came away, again late, but I remember driving down the*** and having to pull over and I just wept. Really wept and felt emotionally drained (participant 9)

One of the nursing home respondents implies that others might think that she cannot cope if she is seen to cry, so she tends to find somewhere to cry alone:

Sometimes I break down in tears…There's been a few residents who I've cried with. A couple of the staff who I've had a cry with. But most of the time I will shut myself away and have that cry…I think I do it so that people think I can cope, I shut myself away… (participant 3)

Campbell[10] describes how the closeness of contact with the patient means a costly mutuality for the nurse. This is illustrated by another respondent from the nursing home who was upset, because she had not been present when a patient she had grown close to had died. She needed to arrange to see the deceased patient to say goodbye as part of her coming to terms with the situation:

We did have one lady die here who I was close to and I went and saw her in the hospital… at rest…I went and saw her because…I was so upset, I'd never said goodbye…I asked my manager at the time and she said I could arrange it just phone up and ask…it did make a difference…I always thought I would never want to do that, I would never want to see someone that's passed away, I'd rather remember them as they were, but actually she would just follow me all the time, you turned around and she was there, so it was such a loss that she suddenly wasn't there (participant 5)

The toll of coping with loss is described as more than psychological, in that emotional exhaustion contributes to physical depletion:

I think sometimes it can take quite a lot out of you without you realising and I just feel quite exhausted sometimes. And you think well I haven't physically done that much today, but you get home from work and you're so tired, you think well emotionally it's been quite a hard day (participant 10)

SUMMARY

As well as sharing details of personal loss in the throes of being interviewed, nurses frequently indicated the emotional challenge of repeated exposure to situations of significant loss in practice. In getting to know their patients over a period of time, the death of a patient was a situation of loss for the nurse as well as the family. Nurses tended to grieve privately in order not to compromise their professional support for bereaved relatives and friends. However, support for nurses is essential if they are to maintain their own spiritual integrity in the face of repeated exposure to the suffering incurred by loss.

REFERENCES

1. James N. Emotional labour: skill and work in social regulation of feelings. *Sociological Review*. 1989; **37**(1): 15–42.

2. McNamara B, Waddell C and Colvin M. Threats to the good death: the cultural context of stress and coping among hospice nurses. *Sociology of Health and Illness*. 1995; **17**(2): 222–44.

3. Bobinac A, Job N, van Exel A, *et al.* Caring for and caring about: disentangling the caregiver effect and the family effect. *J Health Econ*. 2010; **29**(4): 549–56.

4. Campbell A. *Moderated Love: a Theology of Professional Care*. London: SPCK, 1984.

5. Parkes CM *Bereavement: Studies of Grief in Adult Life*. 3rd ed. London: Routledge, 1996.

6. Campbell, op. cit.

7. Davies B and Oberle K. Dimensions of the supportive role of the nurse in palliative care. *Oncology Nursing Forum*. 1990; **17**(1): 87–94.

8. Walter T. *On Bereavement: the Culture of Grief*. Buckingham: Open University Press, 1999.

9. Stroebe M and Schut H. The dual process model of coping with bereavement: rationale and description. *Death Studies*. 1999; **23**: 197–224.

10. Campbell, op. cit.

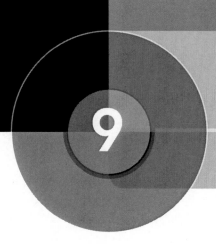

Belonging as the means of nurses coping

9

The rapport between team members and the team and its organization's management is important in developing meaningful relationships and purpose in the work environment. In this sense, right relationships provide a spiritually supportive ambience in the workplace.[1] Belonging to a nursing team is a primary source of support in end of life practice. Team dynamics are therefore particularly important when nurses rely on their peers for support in situations that can be emotionally demanding.[2] Dominant issues of loss differed across practice environments, and this influenced the dynamics of the teams in which nurses belonged and which they looked to for support. Although participants' teams shared the goal of providing holistic care for patients nearing the end of their life, their team cultures differed in the style of support sourced within the teams.

DIFFERENCE IN DOMINANT ISSUES OF LOSS

Hospice nurses associate loss within their working environment primarily with the consequences of dying and death. This is described very factually:

…in the hospice environment it obviously is about death and dying because half of our patients that are admitted die, and all the ones – most of the ones – that are referred to us will die (participant 6)

The irrefutability of loss for patients and relatives was seen to commence with the diagnosis of terminal illness:

I think the loss, the patient's and relatives' loss, starts at diagnosis…being diagnosed with a life-threatening illness or being told that the disease…is terminal… (participant 2)

However, one hospice nurse's response saw a shift in focus, to that of the anticipated loss of a person:

I suppose immediately we think of someone dying…And in terms of the family I suppose the most immediate thing you most quickly think about is them actually losing someone, dying (participant 7)

This issue was raised more strongly in comments by community nurses. As 'guests' in their patients' homes, community nurses work with the family in situ, and perhaps this is why they particularly convey their awareness of the impact of loss on the patient's significant others, as circumstances change both relationships and the need for support. Primary issues of loss were those of relationship and its associated activities, for example:

…the loss of partnership, the companionship, the loss of making decisions, being alone… (participant 9)

The comprehensive nature of loss suffered by those admitted to a nursing home is affirmed by the suggestion that residents have 'lost the lives they have had':

…I mean, people who are coming into a nursing home, first of all they've lost their lives that they've had. You get some people who come here who have quite complex bereavements and…who've lost the people they care about (participant 3)

Loss of their home, above all losses, was considered by one nurse to be more significant to residents than dying:

…loss of family here, because a lot of the people here are here so long and they're so disabled they tend to lose a lot of visitors, some of them never have visitors, it's quite hard to see that, but yes just losing their social thing, their work, if they have been in really quite high-powered jobs they've lost that, they've lost their home. You know I think sometimes that's more of an issue than the fact that they're going to die… (participant 5)

The resultant challenges of communal living are reflected in a comment by a hospice nurse who had previously run a residential home:

And I did see in some cases, particularly those elderly people who were single, what a tremendous amount they had had to give up to come in, and what a huge adjustment they had to make to living in a communal setting, something that they'd never had to do since they were children. And that made a big impression on me, just how much they had had to adjust (participant 2)

Locus of control, as previously mentioned (see Chapter 6), is an aspect of personality theory that describes an individual's tendency to either believe that they are largely in control of their own lives, or that some other agent – such as God, environmental factors or other people – determines their fate.[3] Some have pointed out that there is an assumption that individuals will become more prone to be external in their locus of control as they age.[4] However, residents who chose to remain in their room, the only space within communal living accommodation that they can call their 'own', is an example of one means by which they can retain control over their lives in a situation of loss, rather than comply to invitations of professional carers. Regardless, the importance of encouraging them to emerge and engage in new relationships as a means of coping and avoiding isolation, a major theme in the cause of depression in older nursing home residents,[5] is reflected in the following nurse's experience:

We've had a few people here who, when they first come here, they don't want to come out of their rooms, they don't want people to see them like they are…that they can't get up and walk, they can't do this, and so you try and work with people to try and stop… like…because when somebody gets isolated they become very introvert and very negative because they've…you know what I mean? And it's quite a common thing which can happen to quite a few people, so it's about trying to find them things that will get them out of their rooms (participant 3)

Protocols for addressing care of the dying, adapted for each end of life care practice environment, have been devised and disseminated nationally. These protocols include addressing patients' and relatives' spiritual issues.[6,7]

INFORMAL SUPPORT FOR NURSES WITHIN TEAMS

A shared value system that invests meaning and direction in care is understood to be the key to the ability to work long-term in environments involving recurrent exposure to loss.[8] This shared value system drives work ethos and understanding of what is meant by having done a good job. If this is the case, it is not surprising that most nurses chose to look to their team members for informal support at work, and found this particularly beneficial. Such informal support is often spontaneous, coming from instinctual awareness of need by those giving the support. This is due to their own past experience of similar situations, or their having to cope with current dire circumstances alongside colleagues, so that in that sense they are 'in this together'.

The means and style of support valued was to some extent linked to practice context; for example, nurses working in the hospice environment spoke of the ways in which support was generally available within the team. This was explained by one nurse as being related to the nature of the team. Nurses who are able to 'stay' the course of palliative working environments were considered to collectively imbue an ambience of support, in that support 'bounces off staff' without them needing to ask 'what's the matter?' They also 'look out for staff' who are know to be dealing with complex care needs:

But the team here, they really are excellent…generally speaking, once you start here, you either realize palliative care isn't for you or you stay and there's lots of us that have been here for a long time. And it's something that bounces off the staff and that you know you are in a supportive environment and you don't need to say to somebody, what's the matter? What's happened? You just instinctively know that something isn't right. And by [the] nature of our handovers and getting to know our patients we know – well we don't know but have an idea of – the difficulties that we can encounter with different patients and families and, if a member of staff is looking after a patient with a complex family then we know during the day to look out for them and just to keep an ear open…And…our office, you know, behind closed doors – we let off steam, and we sort of pass things amongst ourselves, you know, to get it off our chests and to get back to a good place (participant 2)

The tendency for the hospice team to 'look out for each other' was reiterated by another respondent, who emphasized the importance of knowing 'what's going on' so that colleagues are protected from being in a difficult situation for too long:

…it certainly is here anyway. It's very supportive and we all know which situations are difficult and we all look out for each other, so we might also…if someone's spent a long time in a difficult situation then someone might take over and give you a break. Yes, and being aware of what's going on. I think people are very good at that here to be honest. Yes, on the whole that's how it works (participant 7)

Description of informal support also reflects what it is they need support with. In having to manage their emotions in the face of patient and relative distress, support within the team is taken to mean ensuring staff are aware of how they feel, and that they have the opportunity to express that in whatever way is most appropriate for them:

…being in touch with your feelings, I think the worst thing you can do in this job is to bury it and just ignore it, you've got to reflect on those feelings and be in touch with those feelings and find ways of expressing them, but quite often because you're a member of staff there's that sense that you've got to be coping and getting on…you can't be showing your feelings to relatives but somehow you do need to do that in an appropriate way and making sure that there is a facility to be able to do that. And I think with staff it's about supporting each other and allowing each other to cry if we need to… (participant 8)

The centrality of a sense of team as a creation of self-empowering support is also reflected by most of the community nurse respondents. Here, 'banter' is the style of communication for a diversity of nurses to share personal 'stuff':

and the girls I think also feel…that we have each other in here and we're quite diverse really, some who're thinking of retiring down to…a staff nurse who's [recently qualified] and has been in community for about a year now. So we're quite diverse but we all have our own experiences, I think we all draw on that. There's a time…you know there's good bantering there and there's lots of personal stuff but I think if there was…I think we're quite perceptive to the team, the team's wants and needs… (participant 9)

Such talk is located 'back at the office' and helps keep troubled feelings in perspective:

…we come back to the office and talk to one another and I think that's a huge benefit, to talk to one another about things and our worries, because it helps to put everything into perspective (participant 10)

The younger members of the team, who had only been working in the community for a year, were aware of the availability of colleague support as a resource to help them cope with the emotional challenges of work:

…I have a great team here so I know that if anything upset or bothered me we could all talk about it… (participant 12)

…talking to colleagues…because they understand…So that generally is how I would do with it if I was ready to talk to anybody (participant 11)

INFORMAL SUPPORT FOR AND BY MEMBERS OF THE WIDER TEAM

Other than informal support within nursing teams, there were a couple of exemplars where nurses provided support for their support workers. One example was a participant in the nursing home who described how informal support is provided for support staff following the death of a resident they have known for a long time. She gives staff the opportunity to choose to express how they feel, including the option to view the deceased resident if they want to say a final goodbye. In addition, she offers her personal support in inviting support workers to help her perform the final act of care in laying the patient out, and perhaps in this way is giving them the opportunity to face any potential fear they may have in dealing with the dead in a supportive setting:

…you try and speak to all the staff if someone dies, and we've had residents that have been here for years, so obviously you've got to give the staff a chance to express how they feel about that, if you're looking after someone for years and then they die, it's picking [that] up isn't it and giving them the opportunity, saying, look if you haven't done this before, if you want to go in and do last offices with me you can, but at the same time you can't force someone to do that, you've got to be sensitive, they maybe might not want to do that. And we have had people die here and they've been waiting to go to the undertakers, we've had loads of staff...go into to the room to say goodbye to them... (participant 5)

The same nurse also valued the thoughtfulness reflected in support offered by her own manager. She had cared for a young man who was dying and whose mother needed a great deal of support. The nurse's manager took the time to ask how she was after dealing with this death and to support her. In this way her account of her experience reflected the cascade of impromptu informal support provided both by her for immediate colleagues and for her by the wider staffing of the nursing home:

The managers are pretty good here, I mean my manager...found time to come and speak to me afterwards and say to me are you ok and to support me (participant 5)

Two respondents also chose specific sources of support that were available informally, but not within their immediate team. The first found Heron's[9] style of organized peer support helpful. This is an arrangement where people meet regularly to help each other develop personally and professionally. It is a self-generating and self-renewing form of support. The respondent in question arranged to participate in peer supervision with a colleague in the nursing home who worked on a different floor, and who she felt had similar values to her own. Meetings appeared to be arranged on an 'as necessary' basis and allowed them both to 'talk things through' and pass any issues 'by each other':

I've got a nurse who I do like peer supervision with, who works upstairs, and we'll meet up. Sometimes we'll have periods where we'll meet once a month and then sometimes we won't have it for a few months. So we meet up together and sort of talk things through...I'd been working here for over a year and obviously you get a lot of stuff going on and I think...I mean it wasn't until I had been here like three or four years that I really started getting to know the staff. But she was a nurse who...if you've got an issue, you'll get together to discuss things like do I need to call a doctor, do I need to do this sort of thing......and you'll pass it by each other. And she was a nurse who seemed to be close to the values that I had (participant 3)

The second respondent who benefited from an additional source of informal support was a member of the community nursing team. She explained that of the six surgeries that she covered, one felt particularly supportive. The surgery in question was founded on a Christian ethos and conveyed the sense of working within a family. The surgery has its own pastor who is available to talk through problems. She very much valued feeling part of this surgery, in just belonging:

One of the surgeries I work for has a very strong Christian foundation and it's like working in a family, so I think I've drawn a lot from there. We have our own pastor, one of the GP's husbands, if we need to, and I've often thought: oh I've got a problem...and I know he's there if I need to talk to him. He's a lovely guy and I've seen him professionally and we go out at Christmas and what-have-you and always think: oh, there is that resource there. But I think it's the…just the general philosophy of the whole of the surgery, only one surgery bearing in mind I've got six to cover. Just that one where I can just go in to that surgery and just phew…and just feel part of being there, belonging, so…I don't feel that in any of the others…whereas this particular surgery I'm talking about is like family, my work family – I have my home family plus my work family (participant 9)

FORMAL SUPPORT FOR NURSES

Formal support does have cost implications, not only in time, in taking staff out of practice situations, but in remuneration for specialist support. One nurse had found a hospice forum in which staff explored actual case studies that involved challenging patient and staff issues particularly helpful in working through things that 'weighed heavily on her mind'. Attendance was voluntary. At interview the respondent's account was very much a reflection on the loss of what had been helpful, which was further evidenced by her seeking to find out why these meetings had stopped:

…it was sort of like they did a one-off group counselling session that was actually run by a counsellor and where you could go and just sort of say…you know, you could say what you found really hard…and it was the psychotherapist who led that from outside the hospice, and it was absolutely…I thought it was really good, I hadn't been here long and I really had some…I was named nurse for this patient who sort of…what is the right word…there were some really big issues there, and I really liked this patient and there was just so many things and it just weighed heavily on my mind…and as a nurse [I] could say 'oh I would like to do this on such-and-such patient' and I did that, and you know it was brilliant!…you then presented your patient with the problems and there were…nurses and social worker, and the doctors used to come…and it was really encouraged, and the psychotherapist…anyway I did think beforehand that it wasn't going to do something but it really did, it just all…it laid everything to rest. And that…stopped and I was told because of finances (participant 1)

Education that facilitates understanding is another potential source of formally accessed support. All but the youngest community nurse had accessed study focused on palliative care. Hospice and nursing home respondents had also participated in specific courses on loss and bereavement. Although a number of participants had achieved specialist graduate qualifications, the majority of courses attended were not accredited, and had been provided by the hospice local to the nurses' work environment. This reflects the ethos of hospice philosophy in educating the wider professional workforce in the principles of end of life care.

It was my choice to do the palliative care course. And if I saw anything that was available…I would feel confident I could go and ask and they would fund it within reason (participant 5)

Only one participant referred to formal support that was obligatory. This form of routine supervision by a manager was not felt to be particularly helpful:

…we have to have supervision at least six times a year, so the deputy manager will sit you down every couple of months and will give you supervision, it's not very good quality (participant 3)

The need for staff to actively seek formal support was exemplified by a situation involving a mentally ill patient admitted to the hospice for a prolonged period. This was difficult for nurses with no formal training in mental healthcare. The respondent refers to the forms of support available to help them cope, and outlines what it was they found particularly difficult to cope with:

We went through a very hard time during the time that he was here. We were supported. We had to seek support at various times from the family support team for ourselves, and we had debriefings, because again we are all individuals and our level of…our coping mechanisms are different, and we were all trying to cope with this one man who was very intelligent and he had been sort of institutionalized nearly all his life and he knew how to manipulate people to satisfy his own needs, his own care needs, and that was extremely difficult for a lot of us, particularly the younger ones, the manipulation (participant 2)

IMPACT OF DIFFERENCE ON SUPPORT WITHIN TEAMS

Difference in dominant issues of loss across practice environments reflects to some extent patient situation in their end of life journey, and consequently the nature and intensity of their care needs. This impacts staffing and nursing team dynamics and the style of sourcing support within teams.

Barnard et al.'s[10] study of palliative nursing implied collegial working involved a shared responsibility, not only for patient care but also in nurses supporting one another. Hospice care is provided primarily for the terminally ill. The ratio of registered nurses to patient numbers is high due to the need for 'intensive care' for patients who are usually admitted for specialists to manage symptoms that have been too challenging for professionals to manage in other environments.[11] Therefore, although situations that the participants faced were at times harrowing, they were never 'alone' in that there were always other registered members of the nursing team on shift and so collegial support was available.

In community care a shift in health policy due to sicker patients living longer[12] has resulted in increasing numbers of patients, and the complexity of their needs associated with end of life care, contributing to an increasing workload. Both patients with advanced chronic disease and terminal illness are cared for at home for longer, rather than being admitted for institutional care. In these circumstances the ratio of registered nurses to patients needs to be robust, but access to support in difficult circumstances is delayed or dependent on catching a colleague 'back at the office' due to logistics leaving the nurse 'alone' while travelling and visiting patients.

In the nursing home environment individuals are almost exclusively elderly and, on admission, may only need supportive care. However, over a period of time, the clients grow more dependent and ultimately require end of life care. In order to manage such a range of need, and remain financially viable, the ratio of registered nurses to clients in this environment was lower, with perhaps one registered nurse managing a team of care assistants on each 'floor' of the nursing home. The culture of support within the team appeared to constitute a tripartite system. Nurses were responsible for supporting support workers who worked on the floor that they were in charge of. Second, there was evidence that nurses supported each other. However, this support was not necessarily immediately available, despite their working in an institutional environment. This was because the limited number and geographical spacing of nurses leaves them 'alone' in practice when facing difficult circumstances. Therefore support is delayed until they are able to ring a colleague at home, or arrange to meet, perhaps for peer supervision. A third facet of support was from the manager outside the immediate nursing team, which included clinical supervision, although this was not considered beneficial. Nicklin's[13] model outlines the three complementary but often contradictory functions of supervision. First, normative function is managerial and focused on delivery of efficient and effective care. Second, formative function is educational and concerns skills maintenance and development, and third, restorative function is supportive and addresses managing and minimising occupational stressors. The purpose of clinical supervision is to sustain the balance between these functions. If supervision was skewed and failed to address restorative functions adequately this may account for why it was not helpful.

SUMMARY

Difference in dominant issues of loss reflects the continuum of end of life care provision, from the supportive environment of a nursing home for those with progressive chronic illness that will render them in need of end of life care in due course, through support that enables those adjusting to losses in the throes of their end of life journey to remain in their own homes (including nursing homes), to intensive care for those patients admitted to a hospice with challenging needs, half of whom are near death. These differences in end of life care settings impact staffing and nursing team dynamics, and consequently the styles of support for nurses within their teams.

REFERENCES

1. Wright SG. Faith, hope, and clarity. *Nursing Standard*. 2002; **17**(6): 22–3.
2. Field D. *Nursing the Dying*. London: Routledge, 1989.
3. Rotter JB. Internal versus external control of reinforcement: a case history of a variable. *American Psychologist*. 1990; **45**(4): 489–93.
4. Aldwin CM and Gilman DF. *Health, Illness and Optimal Ageing*. London: Sage, 2004.

5. Choi NG, Ransom S and Wyllie RJ. Depression in older nursing home residents: the influence of nursing home environmental stressors, coping, and acceptance of group and individual therapy. *Aging and Mental Health*. 2008; **12**(5): 536–47.

6. Thomas K. *Caring for the Dying at Home: Companions on the Journey*. Oxford: Radcliffe Medical Press, 2003.

7. Ellershaw J and Wilkinson S. *Care of the Dying: a Pathway to Excellence*. Oxford: Oxford University Press, 2003.

8. McNamara B, Waddell C and Colvin M. Threats to the good death: the cultural context of stress and coping among hospice nurses. *Sociology of Health and Illness*. 1995; **17**(2): 222–44.

9. Heron J. *The Complete Facilitator's Handbook*. London: Kogan Page, 1999.

10. Barnard A, Hollingum C, Hartfiel B. Going on a journey: understanding palliative care nursing. *International Journal of Palliative Nursing*. 2006; **12**(1): 6–12.

11. Randall F and Downie RS. *The Philosophy of Palliative Care: Critique and Reconstruction*. Oxford: Oxford University Press, 2006.

12. Thomas, op. cit.

13. Nicklin P. A practice-centred model of clinical supervision. *Nursing Times*. 1997; **93**(46): 52–4.

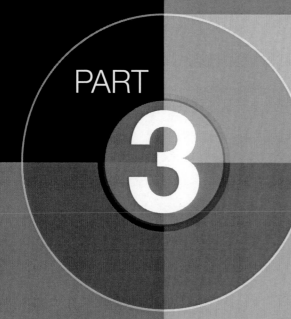

PART 3

THE IMPACT OF PROCESS OF CARE ON NURSES' PROFICIENCY IN SPIRITUAL CARE

Donabedian[1] considers that the 'process' of care constitutes those activities that go on within and between practitioners and patients. In this study, process of care was found to be related directly to patient need. The nature of process in relation to the circumstances of need increased the potential of spiritual development in the nurses themselves.

Spirituality is experiential in nature, and therefore an understanding of this concept tends to be 'caught' rather than taught.[2] Spirituality in healthcare contexts can be promoted in education forums by experiential methods of delivery, and benefit nurses' awareness of what constitutes spiritual care.[3] However, it is in practice environments, where there is an interface with existential issues, that spiritual development is really honed.

The following chapters incorporate descriptions of process that illuminate how participants grow in spiritual maturity and how this growth contributes to their proficiency in spiritual care.

REFERENCES

1. Donabedian A. *The Definition of Quality and Approaches to Assessment*. Ann Arbor, MI: Health Administration Press, 1980.
2. Bradshaw A. Teaching spiritual care to nurses, an alternative approach. *International Journal of Palliative Nursing*. 1997; **3**(1): 51–7.
3. Greenstreet W. *Teaching Spirituality in Nursing* [Dissertation]. Canterbury: Christ Church College, 1996.

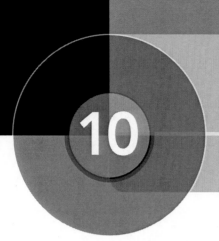

Belief as the pillar of spirituality

10

How an understanding of belief is achieved varies. In applying our consciousness to search for an understanding of how and why things happen, if we come to uphold a belief even if there is no proof then we are said to make an explicit profession of faith.[1] If our search for the truth is more a matter of conceptual analysis or thinking about thinking, then we are destined to arrive at a philosophical conclusion to our quest.[2] Published literature already asserts the significance of nurses clarifying their own spiritual stance.[3,4,5] Spiritual awareness that enables nurses to differentiate between patient and personal spiritual issues is particularly important if they are to support patients asking 'ultimate' questions as they face real life and death issues of existence. Research participants associated the term 'spirituality' with meaning and purpose in life. Their experience reflects a pattern in the development of belief, the outcome of which, whether religious or non-religious, is a significant resource in regulating distress associated with loss as well as shaping coping strategies.

MEANING AND PURPOSE

In a number of ways nurses associated spirituality as a concept concerned with meaning and purpose in life, for example:

...just the meaning of life, what is the meaning and purpose of us being here other than to do the things that we do physically on a daily basis (participant 5)

Life's meaning was seen to involve a search, a journey of discovery:

Another way of looking at spirituality is that search for meaning isn't it? I think Frankl talks about the search for meaning, and I think we are all in that search...the journey of discovery (participant 8)

Encouraging patients to find something that gives them a sense of worth in their lives helps preserve feelings of purpose. Worth contributes to a sense of value and so this strategy is also one of generating and/or sustaining hope:[6]

...from experience, different people have different things that they find important in their lives and it's about encouraging them to do...or to find something that helps them to feel as though their lives are worthwhile (participant 3)

Existential questioning fundamentally focuses on 'why' things have happened.[7] Such questions can create considerable suffering[8] as patients or relatives struggle to understand the meaning and purpose of what has happened or is happening to them. One respondent described a scenario in which a 50-year-old patient was trying to make sense of her situation; having sustained an injury that had left her totally paralysed, she was angry and wanting to know:

...why did they leave me like this? (participant 4)

Such a question can be interpreted as either a question of causality or a question of meaning.[9] The nurse responded to the question as one of causality. Her response largely reflected the good intent of the emergency team in recovering the patient from unconsciousness:

...you'd sort of go back to basics and you'd say – when you were unconscious and you went into A&E and you (had) fallen off the balcony or downstairs or whatever it was, they tried to do good, because the rule is to do good not to do harm. And they tried to do good and the fact you've ended up like this wasn't the intention and they didn't know that when they brought you back to life (participant 4)

However, the question was evidently one that reflected the patient's struggle to find meaning, as her anger was still not abated when she left the nursing home after community care had been arranged:

She went away nursing her rage and her anger... (participant 4)

Questions of meaning are rarely answerable, but understanding helps.[10] A beneficial approach was reflected in one nurse's response to questions of untimely loss. He was self-aware in acknowledging that he may come to certain answers himself about such questions, but these may well not be right for someone else:

...being there, that's really all you can do, you can't say anything can you? The moment you say something it's a platitude and if you think you've got the answers you're in the wrong job basically. You know, you've got to admit there aren't any answers to certain things. And you may have certain answers for yourself but they may not be right for someone else… (participant 8)

Fulfilment achieved through enjoyment of life reflects a psycho-spiritual perception of meaning and purpose in life. Fredrickson[11] suggests that positive emotions such as happiness broaden our thought-action repertoire and help us build psychological resource which can be drawn on at other times, and in different emotional states. Our psychological resources impact our ability to fulfil our life's purpose. Even records of history and ancient philosophy associate happiness with well-being, and claim that when we make full use of our cognitive capacities we are closest to our God-given function.[12,13] One nurse's understanding of spirituality reflects this view:

…it's what makes up your individual world. Things that make you happy, things that interest you, things you get enjoyment out of life that gives you a fulfilled life (participant 12)

RELIGIOUS BELIEF

When asked to talk about what they understood by the term 'spirituality', most participants shared a little of their personal history or story. Many had been socialized into practising a religion within their family culture, and, in sharing these details they implied an association of the term 'spirituality', initially at least, with religious belief. Although they were compliant to their family's religious practice as children, in adolescence and young adulthood most had questioned or strayed from their introduction to religion. However, a number had returned to their faith, albeit with a different perspective; it had been important for them to establish their own belief. Culliford's[14] consideration of a German study by Maria Bindl suggests that this pattern is not unusual. Findings from thousands of drawings on religious themes by Christian children indicated a developmental sequence that reflects a potential decline and then return to spiritual awareness. Initially God is experienced simply, in a one-to-one relationship with the child. Then, as imagination and fantasy are reduced by the ability to reason, their personal experience of God falls into a decline, which is accelerated as their preoccupation with self increases. However, for some, spiritual awareness seems to return in their late teens when they consciously endeavour to seek transcendence.

Participant one, for example, had felt positive about her intense religious upbringing when she was a child. She was taught to believe that the Bible was the exact word of God. She read the Bible and prayed every day, prayer was said at every meal, she attended church twice on Sundays and went to Sunday school when young and religious groups for teenagers later. Her laughter, when describing the duration of compliance in not questioning what she had been taught until she was about 18, seemed to suggest her surprise that it had taken her so long. Although questioning resulted in her 'turning her back', particularly on going to church, she describes the birth of her first child, nearly a decade later, as the moment of certainty in knowing God exists. She has searched but still not found the right church for regular attendance, although she has regained a sense of feeling positive in knowing for herself the existence of God:

> I…was brought up in a strict…protestant environment. Which, when I was a child, I thought of very positively…and I suppose I didn't really question too many things until I was, I don't know, 18 or 19…there was a time when I turned my back to a degree on religion, certainly as far as going to church is concerned…when I had my first child I was 28, so I think I had turned my back for about 8 years by then, I remember the moment he was born I thought, God exists! I remember that. And then think perhaps not going to church, but certainly for myself personally sort of changing and, what shall I say, feeling for myself the existence of God and sort of being more positive…I consider myself a Christian but it's certainly sort of very different from the way I was brought up (participant 1)

Similarly, another respondent conveys the need to find for herself what she had already been taught:

> (Christian faith)…was kind of something I was brought up with but then moved away from and then chose it back for myself. So it's kind of been very much sort of part of my life but it's also something that, having had it put there, I've then gone away and found it for myself (participant 7)

This search for a personal interpretation of belief is evident even in those who have not strayed from religious practice in their youth:

> I think that's changed over my lifetime, I think I used to…as a child I was brought up with quite a strong framework of religion, a Baptist background. My father was a minister of the religion. So I had a very sort of structured framework for my spirituality, and I guess my spirituality was attached to that faith and belief. But as I've grown older, gradually it has become more nebulous really, I guess. More…sort of…I think your religious framework is still quite important to your spirituality but spirituality is greater, it's bigger than the religious framework. And so I think I've described…when I was a child, that I had very deep roots. Those roots are still there, but the branches are slightly different, you know, the outward appearance is slightly different. So my sense of spirituality has changed enormously because of that (participant 8)

As the granddaughter of a Congregational minister, and daughter of an atheist father, one participant persevered in finding her own belief in the face of contradiction. Her account clearly conveyed her sense of 'arrival' when she found a non-conformist church:

I had a grandfather who was…a Congregational minister…I grew up in the manse as my father was in the army…My father was an atheist…He really was anti-God…deep down I always knew there was something bigger than me…I sort of dipped into what I called traditional religion, you know, Anglican church, singing in the choir, as a child – always with my father's disapproval. And then when…I'd just qualified as a nurse, I went to see Billy Graham…I went forward and I've never looked back. And he's a personal saviour of mine and I live the life, a non-conformist church… (participant 4)

NON-RELIGIOUS BELIEF

Outside of comment that was theistic in its reference to God or the religious,[15] most interviewees did give further account of their understanding of the meaning of spirituality that conveyed a non-religious perspective. Connection with another person is not uncommon as a descriptor of an aspect of spirituality,[16,17] but the ways in which that connection is described can vary, for example connection with another person was described as a meeting of souls:

So it's really making that connection with that person and acknowledging that person is a human being just like yourself, with an amazing amount of history behind them, just like you have, and that somehow your two souls have come together and there's a connection there. I guess that, in reality, is what I see as spirituality in…practice (participant 8)

Being a person exists essentially in relationship and entails communication.[18] Traits of humanity, such as the ability to think, believe and have morals, allow us to make choices.[19] Therefore, in choosing how we are with and how we treat others we contribute to our growth in 'becoming' who we are as a person. In this way description of non-religious spirituality also infers that spirituality is a constituent of personhood:

…I think it's about how you think and how you are and what you believe in. And I don't mean religious-wise, I mean morals…and how you treat people (participant 10)

The shared set of beliefs, values and behaviour patterns learnt within our culture influence how we understand our experience.[20] It is not surprising, therefore, that culture is mentioned as influencing our understanding of spirituality. In addition, spirituality is described as inherent within us. This is not dissimilar to McColl's[21] understanding of spirituality as a human characteristic, our ability to experience and incorporate spirit into our lives. However, McColl[22] believes that it is spirit that exists independently 'out there', and not 'lots of spirituality', as described in the following:

…a belief, a part of oneself. From cultural, from upbringing, anything that's passed on…something that you kind of believe in yourself. Something, that's just personal to yourself; there's lots of spirituality out there but it's something that's inherent in yourself (participant 9)

Spirituality was associated by one nurse with being 'open', and without 'set agendas', in contrast to religions, which are bound by dogma. She does not reject religions outright, but believes that they each may have something to offer and so provide an eclectic understanding of faith. The shift from a collective view of religion to finding meaning for the 'self' is reflected in New Age philosophy. MacLaren[23] describes this philosophy as having its roots in theosophy, which is eclectic in that it includes Hindu, Buddhist and pagan theories. In this sense, the following description of spirituality supports New Age philosophy:

…I would say if I'm perfectly honest! I am quite open-minded, I certainly don't follow a strict religious faith. I never have done from childhood and I can't see that I'll ever be inspired by one set of faith, I like different things from different faiths and don't like rules laid down by religion, it's definitely the spiritual side rather than set agendas (participant 5)

This personal sense of spirituality was illustrated by reference to places of worship and natural environments as sources of inspiration:

You know, if I go to Canterbury Cathedral I find that very inspirational and it is a very powerful place and has got some presence about it but, you know, again if I'm out in the countryside or, even when I was little in Devon and Dartmoor, I find that quite spiritual, especially like the prehistoric stone circles, and the faith of people thousands and thousands of years ago inspires me probably more than faith of a lot of people today (participant 5)

Examples of non-religious activities that might provide a source of spiritual fulfilment involved physical engagement with nature; digging the garden has a preparatory association with growth and snowboarding a means of enjoying the very challenge presented by the elements:

So for some that might be religion and God, for some it might be digging the garden, for some it might be snowboarding (participant 6)

This participant's own source of fulfilment was non-religious; she described her family as the source of the meaning and purpose in her life:

Well I think for me, again, it would be my family – they're the thing that gives me meaning and purpose and encourage me when things are bad or I'm having a stressful time, yes, that's what I would say (participant 6)

There was uncertainty in differentiating between religious and non-religious spiritual issues by one nurse, who describes the dividing line as 'blurred'.

> The thing is I think often the dividing line is blurred. So I'm not absolutely sure about some things, specifically sort of non-religious (participant 1)

Although this participant had largely rejected her strict religious upbringing, her more liberal approach to faith did not appear to engender an understanding of non-religious spirituality. Her practice experience of seeing the pastoral role of the Hospice Chaplain as able to address the wider remit of spirituality as well as the religious needs of patients appears to have resulted in an understanding that any difference is a theoretical distinction.

> ...he (the Hospice Chaplain) is very good also for non-religious spiritual care. So perhaps there isn't that much...there is a theoretical distinction, but...anyway (participant 1)

BELIEF AS A RESOURCE TO 'REGULATE DISTRESS'

Belief is linked to faith by one respondent in attributing a reason to why things happen:

> Faith is a belief that all things happen for a reason. There is a reason, there is a point to our existence (participant 5)

Most participants had had their beliefs tested by experiences in either their current or past practice environments. In different ways the existential question 'why?' was raised by respondents who found it difficult to find the 'reason' for some things happening.

Global dilemmas, and the sudden randomness of loss by a colleague at work were given as examples of situations that fuelled 'doubt':

> I think if you see really bad news, whether it's a world event like terrorism or something horrible, it's very hard to have any faith in anything you know. I do feel you just think it's so horrible you can't see any good or reason to why that should happen. Or people that are born and are starving and you think, why is this? And is there an afterlife...even things at work, we had one of the girls here lost her husband yesterday, completely out of the blue... you just think why?...it's just sad...and I think at those times I do doubt things, I do to be honest. It is very hard to see a positive side or reason for that to happen (participant 5)

Similarly, several nurses reflected on past practice experiences in which they had been challenged by caring for young people who were dying. Societal expectation is one that associates dying and death with old age and chronic ill health. Consequently, dying in youth within western society is considered untimely, and often engenders a sense of struggle in those trying to make sense of such situations,[24] for example:

> …I suppose it's easier to accept somebody who…either has a chronic illness or has a terminal illness if they're older, but if they're younger I think it doesn't seem fair. So I think that's where I sort of struggle a little bit (participant 12)

Untimely death tends to create more anger,[25] and this is evident in one respondent's use of the term 'stolen' when referring to death of the young, hence implying an almost unlawful, illegitimate event. He is also reminded of his own mortality in reviewing his own age in relation to that of the young person dying:

> …I worked in a unit there with HIV and AIDS and in the early days there weren't the antivirals and young people were dying very young, you know. And that feels as if someone's been stolen away and that's really tough. And I find that tough with young people, if someone younger than me dies it really hits home, you know, it shouldn't be happening (participant 8)

Bruce and Schultz[26] describe resilience as involving skills that control anxiety and the perception of unremitting emotional pain. The resilience of her own youth is suggested as the means by which one nurse coped with the intensity of loss of young children in her early professional career. However, she goes on to imply that she did not 'escape' the impact of these experiences:

> Working with young children who have life-threatening orthopaedic conditions and malignant tumours; babies with malignant tumours. At the time I think they distressed me but because I was young and resilient I took them in my stride, but looking back I realize how saddened and how…distressing they were. And then experiences like that have left an impression with me through my nursing career (participant 2)

There were a number of examples of nurses comparing the dying patient's age with their own, but only one who explicitly spoke of a raised awareness of personal mortality. She identifies the loss of a whole series of potential expectations that the family will have to face in losing one of its young members. Such losses are described as non-finite in that the loss is continuous and reviewed over time; for example, parents may review their loss of having been grandparents when they are shown photographs of others' grandchildren.[27] Her comment conveys the difficulty she envisages for the family coping with this loss of expectation and implies a tacit awareness of non-finite loss:

> …in my previous job…and dealing with young people and obviously that's always a tragedy, and it's very upsetting for us as professionals, especially when somebody's young

and it's all of a sudden and it hits the family and how are they going to cope, and their future, looking to a future without that person growing up and getting older or having family or whatever, you know, all those things that a person should be able to have if that's what they choose, it's just taken away. And you know dealing with that from an individual and a professional point of view is quite difficult because...you know, I'm a nurse, I have to support you, but at the same time you're realising your own mortality as well... (participant 12)

The transactional model of stress and coping describes stressful events as those appraised by the individual as a challenge.[28] In this way, a situation that is particularly stressful for one individual is not for another. Some respondents found they were challenged in situations where the family circumstances of the person suffering an untimely death were close to their own family circumstances. One respondent found herself reflecting that it 'could happen to me':

Sometimes you have people come in and die who are younger than you, or they've got young children or it's just been a difficult situation, I think sometimes then you think, oh that could happen to anybody, that could happen to me, how do I deal with it? (participant 7)

Another respondent was completely caught out by her emotional response to one situation. In trying to make sense of why this happened, and why it stayed with her for so long, she reflects on how she was almost putting herself in the patient's position in worrying about how it would be for her own family in those circumstances:

I can only think of one time when I didn't cope...I remember that did stay with me a long time because I had never been that emotional, and I just wondered if it was because of the youth of the family, and thinking, you know, mine were around about the same age and how would it be...you know, it was almost putting me in the position of the patient that had gone, you know, that...the loss, the whole disruption of life through loss, and how would they ever cope and how did that child cope without her mum, and I was reasoning with myself, and I was thinking, no she's got...older siblings...and her dad's great and she'll be fine and...not...worrying about her (participant 9)

Aranda[29] supports the idea that coping in challenging situations is achieved by anything the nurse does to regulate the distress.[30] Respondents gave a number of examples of how their own beliefs help them cope in this way. Belief provides a means of 'processing' situations of loss, a coming to terms with things happening for a reason:

...my own beliefs as well, that's important, because obviously that helps me to sort of process it and think well, ok...it's happened for a reason... (participant 12)

Although faith can fulfil the search for life's meaning and provide a reason for living, a veritable 'rock to stand on', one respondent explained that things happen in the world that 'rub' so 'hard' against that faith, that it becomes refined over time to a point where faith is associated with embracing uncertainty.

> …I think it was Nietzsche who said that he who has a why to live for can cope with almost any how. So to have some reason to live for is very important, and your faith can bring that, and give you a certain rock to stand on…But then there's the flipside to that, if you have got a faith and things happen in the world that rub against that faith hard, it can really be very difficult to handle that. And I certainly found that in my work, it's opened up all sorts of questions about my faith, about my beliefs, and those as the years have gone on have been refined tremendously. I think that's just part of growing up anyhow, to be honest…some of the things I've seen and some of the experiences I've had through all that have knocked me and knocked my faith and made me really have to reflect and rethink and come to new understandings and that's quite painful sometimes…I think it's just arriving at that point where you just have to embrace uncertainty really, you can't say anything is black or white (participant 8)

Similarly, faith is seen as a resource in helping with the acceptance of what we do not know:

> …I don't call myself religious but I am a Christian…there's an awful lot we don't know, we're not supposed to know, that we just have to believe in. And I have that belief (participant 2)

Acceptance not only included that 'things…happen' but also that they may be pre-destined as part of a 'big plan':

> …but I believe there's a big plan for everybody and everybody's part is probably charted to a certain extent and you have to accept some things are going to happen (participant 10)

Compassion is described by Bierhoff[31] as a concern for the suffering of others that makes you want to help them. One respondent's comment inferred the link between faith and compassion when dealing with challenging situations. Faith supports compassion by generating a personal resource in the nurse, in that compassionate understanding promotes tolerance of difficulty in others:

> I think my faith teaches me you have got to forgive and be understanding towards them, especially if somebody's going through a difficult time. They might not behave in the way they normally behave, so you just need to be understanding (participant 10)

PHILOSOPHICAL BELIEF AS A COPING STRATEGY

Many nurses have developed a personal philosophy that helps them cope with repeated exposure to situations of loss. There was some suggestion that coping philosophies were linked to particular personal qualities necessary to survive in end of life care environments. One suggestion was that individuals drawn to nursing as a profession had a tendency for particular traits that supported stoicism, that were strengthened further in being a nurse. The challenges of nursing are seen to demand that you 'keep going' and do not get 'upset all of the time'. The primary focus is outwards, towards others, family and patients who need support. Historically there were no formal means of support and getting upset may have been considered 'a bit of a weakness':

> And part of it, I think, is that sort of stoical nurse type thing – I think you have those traits that's why you choose nursing as a profession and then it reinforces them. Especially I think if you qualified when I did, more than 20 years ago. That was reinforced. But nowadays it's much more acceptable if a nurse gets upset or finds things difficult, but sort of 20 years ago you just had to get on with it because you didn't have supervision and it was probably seen as being a bit weak if you got upset, and you just kept going. So I think you have those tendencies, which is what makes you become a nurse. And then the nursing profession, which makes things hard for itself, reinforces them…but it's a case of, you know, you're dealing with horrible things and death and dying at times, so it's no good getting upset all the time, and there are times when you do, but generally you're there to support the families and the patients so you have to keep going even at times when you feel you really don't want to (participant 6)

In a study by Eley et al.[32] exploring temperament and character traits in nurses and nursing students, outcomes were congruent with a profession still requiring persistence, self-directedness, cooperativeness, dedication and warmth. Therefore the shift from a stoic response to expression of feelings in the face of emotional challenge may be more a matter of a shift in the wider culture of 'Englishness' than in nursing culture itself.

Coping was also attributed to life skills that had come with experience. Eley et al.[33] found that those of middle age, regardless of whether they were nurses or nursing students, scored highest in persistence as a trait of temperament and tended to be reliable and tolerant in character. Therefore, as the middle-aged nursing students will have had less professional experience than the middle-aged nurses in Eley et al.'s[34] study, the life skills referred to below are likely to be as much to do with life experience as that of nursing:

> Because often I will think how do I go on to the next visit having been there at a death or dealt with bereavement or, you know, loss if you like…and I think that only comes with life skills, to be honest, I don't think it's anything you can teach people (participant 9)

One specific means of coping in a situation of loss is described as a comparison of loss; the nurses' loss paling into insignificance in relation to the loss suffered by the patient and relatives:

Yes, you're there [to support families and patients]…yes. Because however bad it is for you, it's not as bad as it is for them (participant 6)

A similar strategy used to cope with challenging emotional situations was bearing in mind that it was the person who was actually suffering who 'owned' the loss. In addition, focusing on the positive outcomes of support offered to patients helps the nurse cope in situations of loss:

A lot of the time, if you can do something to help, or if you can't change the situation you can do something to help them through it or, you know, you can facilitate something that they want doing. That gets you through it because you've done what you can, done something positive and it worked out well. Sometimes situations are very, very sad and there's no getting away from it, no getting around it, nothing you can do about it, you come out of a room and you cry and then you talk…we talk amongst ourselves, and then you get on with it. Because it is a very sad sometimes, you kind of bear in mind it's not your personal loss. It's…just being there for someone else and I think you know if nothing ever got to you, you probably wouldn't be human. But it's not the same as being that person who is actually suffering that loss, you know it's upsetting at the time, but you go away and you can talk through it or go away and do something else, and it's their life not yours so…it's how you deal with it when its all the time (participant 7)

Similarly, focusing on the sense of achievement that comes from doing what the patient wanted was important.

But I…strangely when everything goes right, even though they have died, you actually feel a sense of achievement that you've done it right, you've done what they wanted… (participant 10)

SUMMARY

Belief is a spiritual resource in life's search for meaning and purpose. Questions of meaning are rarely answerable, but understanding the need for such questions helps. Participants implied their association of religion with spirituality, but also included non-religious perspectives of spirituality in their accounts, such as connection with another person, being 'open' and that spirituality is impacted by culture. The difference between religious and non-religious spirituality was described by one nurse as 'blurred'. Situations of untimely death were particularly testing for participants. When the family situation of the patient was close to their own, nurses found it difficult to make sense of their feelings and emotions. However, personal belief and philosophy impacted their aptitude for spiritual care in challenging situations in that it provided a means of nurses accepting or processing loss, whether reliant on being stoical, or focusing on getting care delivery 'right'. Nurses' accounts of their experiences have identified a potential need that education should not only emphasize the importance of nurses' awareness of their own spirituality but also the benefit of a more thorough understanding of belief imbued in practice. Timmins[35] shares this concern; in a self-reporting survey used to collect data based on nurses' views of spirituality, she found that much of nurses' ability to provide responsive spiritual care was based upon their own personal experience, due to the lack of specific education facilitating a broadening of perspective.

REFERENCES

1. Polanyi M. *Science, Faith and Society*. Oxford: Oxford University Press, 1946.
2. Hankinson J. *The Bluffer's Guide to Philosophy*. London: Oval, 2005.
3. Burnard P. The spiritual needs of atheists and agnostics. *Professional Nurse*. 1988; December: 130–2.
4. Cornette K. For whenever I am weak, I am strong… *International Journal of Palliative Nursing*. 1997; **3**(1): 6–13.
5. Greenstreet W. Spiritual wellbeing and spiritual distress. In: Greenstreet W, editor. *Integrating Spirituality in Health and Social Care: Perspectives and Practical Approaches*. Oxford: Radcliffe Publishing, 2006, 32–46.
6. Flemming K. The meaning of hope to palliative care patients. *International Journal of Palliative Nursing*. 1997; **3**(1): 14–18.
7. Peberdy A. Spiritual care of dying people. In: Dickinson D, Johnson M and Samson Katz J, editors. *Death, Dying and Bereavement*. London: Open University Press/Sage, 2000, 73–81.
8. McLeod DL and Wright LM. Living the as-yet unanswered: spiritual care practices in family systems nursing. *Journal of Family Nursing*. 2008; **14**(1): 118–41.
9. Fredriksson L. Modes of relating in caring conversation: a research synthesis on presence, touch and listening. *Journal of Advanced Nursing*. 1999; **30**(5): 1167–76.
10. McLeod and Wright, op. cit.
11. Fredrickson B. The role of positive emotions in positive psychology: the broaden-and-build theory of positive emotions. *American Psychologist*. 2001; **56**(3): 218–26.
12. Mohan K. Eastern perspectives and implications for the West. In: Jewell A, editor. *Ageing, Spirituality and Well-Being*. London: Jessica Kingsley, 2004, 161–79.
13. Scoffham S, Barnes J. Happiness matters: towards a pedagogy of happiness and well being. *The Curriculum Journal*. 2011; **22**(4): 535–48.
14. Culliford L. *The Psychology of Spirituality: An Introduction*. London: Jessica Kingsley, 2011.
15. McSherry W. *The Meaning of Spirituality and Spiritual Care within Nursing and Health Care Practice*. London: Quay, 2007.
16. Burkhardt MA. Spirituality: an analysis of the concept. *Holistic Nursing Practice*. 1989; **3**(3): 69–77.
17. Twycross R. *Introducing Palliative Care*. Oxford: Radcliffe Medical Press, 1999.
18. Habgood J. *Being a Person: Where Faith and Science Meet*. London: Hodder & Stoughton, 1998.
19. Williams R. *Grace and Necessity: Reflections on Art and Love*. London: Morehouse, 2005.
20. Speck P. Cultural issues in palliative care for non-cancer patients. In: Addington-Hall J and Higginson I, editors. *Palliative Care for Non-cancer Patients*. Oxford: Oxford University Press, 2001.

21. McColl AM. Spirit, occupation and disability. *Canadian Journal of Occupational Therapy.* 2000; **67**(4): 217–28.

22. Ibid.

23. MacLaren J. A kaleidoscope of understandings: spiritual nursing in a multi-faith society. *Journal of Advanced Nursing.* 2004; **45**(5): 457–62.

24. Sheldon F. *Psychosocial Palliative Care.* Cheltenham: Stanley Thornes, 1997.

25. Ibid.

26. Bruce J and Schultz C. *Nonfinite Loss and Grief.* London: Jessica Kingsley, 2001.

27. Ibid.

28. Lazarus RS and Folkman S. *Stress Appraisal and Coping.* New York: Springer, 1984.

29. Aranda S. The cost of caring. In: Payne S, Seymour J and Ingleton C, editors. *Palliative Care Nursing: Principles and Evidence for Practice.* Maidenhead: McGraw/Open University Press, 2008, 573–90.

30. Folkman S. Positive psychological states and coping with severe illness. *Social Science and Medicine.* 1997; **45**(8): 1207–221.

31. Bierhoff H-W. The psychology of compassion and prosocial behaviour. In: Gilbert P, editor. *Compassion Conceptualisations: Research and Use in Psychology.* London: Routledge, 2005.

32. Eley D, Eley R, Young L *et al.* Exploring temperament and character traits in nurses and nursing students in large regional area of Australia. *Journal of Clinical Nursing.* 2010; **20**: 563–70.

33. Ibid.

34. Ibid.

35. Timmins F. Nurses' views of spirituality and spiritual care in the republic of Ireland. *Journal for the Study of Spirituality.* 2013; **3**(2): 123–39.

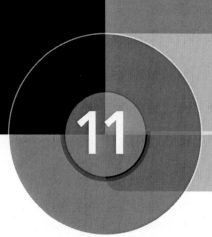

Being a 'spiritual carer'

11

…tasks have got to be done and they feel as if they're getting in the way, but actually it's the way you do those that brings in the spirituality (participant 8)

Participant responses conveyed an understanding of the significance of particular ways of behaving towards others, in order to develop trust and rapport, as a conduit of spiritual care. In this way, choosing how they are with, and how they treat others, contributes to their own growth in being a spiritual carer. The style of relationship between nurse and patient that results is in itself a spiritual resource. Establishing rapport involved a variety of approaches and activities that included exploratory conversation, documented guidance, intuitive sensing, supportive presence and active listening. Time was also an issue. Occasionally, despite opportunity, patients who seemed troubled chose not to share their concerns. In establishing a relationship that is open to sharing patients' suffering, participants also indicated their need for self-care, and the value of personal replenishment to maintain their own spiritual well-being.

THE VALUE OF RAPPORT

Establishing a rapport is considered fundamental to a relationship of trust. Trust opens communication by those who are vulnerable of significant matters which, if shared, can facilitate coping:

…well, after they get to know you, but even sometimes, for them to be able to talk to you to express how they're feeling, worries, anxieties, to allow them to do that and I guess to make them comfortable that they can do that… (participant 11)

Communication that reflects spiritual caring is described by Morse *et al.*[1] as a style that to some extent pre-dates professional learning. Reflexive responses are patient-focused and triggered by the emotional insight of the carer. The emotional involvement reflects the fact that the carer is 'connected' and able to identify with the sufferer. Such care is described by James[2] as emotional labour, and demands both strength and energy. Immersion in another's reality results in sharing the experience or 'burden' of suffering:

I myself like to think, and I'm sure other people do that as well, that if you have built up a rapport with people that they might well, you know, sort of talk to you, and sometimes even just talking about it or expressing fears and anxieties is sort of partly helping, if not completely, but yes…just sharing the burden, but I think that happens when people feel they have a rapport with you (participant 1)

EXPLORATORY CONVERSATION

To care for another is to value them. In order to provide care it is important to know something of the situation and needs of those requiring care. Caring conversation is a means of exploring the patient's personal suffering.[3] Several participants considered conversation the most natural means of conducting an assessment of spiritual need. Metaphor was used by participant 8 to convey his intuitive unease in using illustrative questions set out in a more formal assessment document rather than conversation, in that it did not 'ring right':

And I suppose you've got to start somewhere. But I find that when you're in with someone, to start asking those sort of questions as a spiritual assessment just doesn't ring right with me. I think you assess someone's spirituality by being with them for a period of time, and it's from the conversations that flow from that. But you, I think if you've got a sheet which is a 'spiritual assessment' and you have got to fill it in during admission and you feel as if you've got to ask these questions, it feels very forced and very artificial. Whereas if you've had two or three shifts with this person and look after them and had conversations, from that you can elicit a lot more information which sort of defines where they are coming from spiritually (participant 8)

Others also prefer conversation to questioning as an effective means of understanding how patients feel, their beliefs and what it is they need, for example:

I don't think you should underestimate talking to a patient about how they feel, their beliefs, what they want, because you find out far more by doing that than just by asking them a few questions. If I need to go and find out about a patient I try not to go in and just ask them questions, you might have to start off initially with asking a couple of questions, but you then let them talk and you learn far more about them that way than just asking questions (participant 10)

In their classification of need, Ewles and Simnett[4] describe a felt need as one that an individual has identified, where there is some difference from their norm. In engaging with patients, being supportive and trying to understand how they feel, participant 11 enables patients to move felt need on to expressed need.

…there's more to nursing than just literally going in and doing a task, there's emotional support, there's…you know…understanding their feelings and letting the person talk about things…being concerned about the person as a whole…from patients themselves volunteering that information (participant 11)

USE OF DOCUMENTED GUIDANCE

Ritualistic practices are described by McLeod and Wright[5] as those prescribed for all accessing a service. They acknowledge the importance of an appropriate attitude by the nurse performing the ritual, but argue that, performed thoughtfully, they can open space for reading spiritual need and in the process promote healing. Participant 9 felt a written document including guiding questions was useful in initiating a spiritual assessment. She indicates in her use of metaphor the importance of accepting the patient's response if the 'barrier is up' and they do not wish to discuss this aspect of care further; in indicating the need for assessment to be ongoing, and not 'parked' because the patient's needs change and they may later need 'something to latch onto' for support:

…sometimes it's hard to do this assessment without the documentation, so I think if you hit the documentation and you get to an area of spirituality, cultural beliefs etc, I think you just ask the question, what's on the document, and I think, you know, following on your questioning would be whatever the patient replies. 'I don't believe in anything', 'I have no spiritual belief,' you know, no…they don't want to go there. So that's quite difficult. But you've got to abide by that, that's their wishes, they don't wish to discuss anything and they don't want to go down that line. So that's it, the barrier's up if you like…I think it changes, as you're nursing people I think the assessment's not all parked, it changes…it's a progress, it changes and maybe you'll get to a point in the last few days where the patient will ask, where they will just throw up a question where you might think well maybe they do need a priest or a vicar or some kind of something to latch onto (participant 9)

INTUITIVE SENSING

Confidence and familiarity are linked by participant 10 to patients being comfortable and being willing to talk. However, she goes on to imply that sometimes she intuitively is aware of a need in people without being able to give an account of why this is other than 'you just sense things':

…through talking to people and being quite open with them, letting them lead the way when you're talking to them about things. Gaining their confidence really, because then they're more comfortable around you and they'll talk about things and then once you get to know somebody you can recognize things in them easier than you can a stranger.

But then sometimes you can just pick things up, you just sense things, a need in people, without understanding why you sense things you just do (participant 10)

Similarly, a hospice respondent used the phrases 'you sort of sense' and 'intuitively recognize' in relation to being aware of spiritual need:

I think sort of talking to people or being with them, you can sort of sense spiritual things and often…or people might say things to you and obviously not usually sort of direct… sometimes people tell you directly about a spiritual need, but not always. Where I then sort of – I don't know – intuitively recognize spiritual needs (participant 1)

She went on to describe a patient scenario to illustrate when she had found intuitive 'sensing' occurred, but could not find words to further explain the experience of 'sensing' another's spiritual need:

I don't know if I can really explain to you. I remember a young person being here, in her early 30s, who was terminally ill and she was just, though I suppose you could just imagine anybody in a state like that, it's obviously sad and depressing because nobody wants to be terminally ill and in their early 30s. But we used to talk, obviously talking about nursing care things and sort of needs, so let's call it physical needs that had to be met, or nursing care needs. But there was always…I could always sense that there were far greater things on this person's mind, and I don't know if I can describe it any better than that, just this sensing (participant 1)

SUPPORTIVE PRESENCE

Verbal communication is not always considered necessary in establishing a rapport, but the supportive presence of just sitting with a patient may induce sufficient confidence to enable them to begin to share their worst fears. Pettigrew[6] suggests that the healing power of vulnerability comes from the nurse's willingness to stay with the patient, rather than try to say or do the right thing:

…sometimes patients just don't want to talk about things or perhaps find it too difficult… and sometimes just sitting with them. And then I have experienced myself that… sometimes you don't need to say anything and sometimes you can just sit with a patient and nothing has to be said or will be said, but…sometimes, you gain somebody's confidence and then they might sort of talk about things, or just express their despair or just express that they just don't know what to do (participant 1)

ACTIVE LISTENING

Participant 8 uses analogy and metaphor to describe our shared humanity as a 'journey' in which 'the world unfolds in front of us'. Being alongside people at the end of their life's journey is seen as one way of giving spiritual care. The process of active listening is one of consciously paying attention, and searching for meaning and understanding to interpret what is being said.[7] It is active listening that both facilitates identifying patient spiritual need and provides a means of giving spiritual care:

> I think it's the whole of comforting, you know we're all on a journey and we're all sort of on a journey of discovery I suppose, as the world unfolds in front of us, and in some ways, every day is a brand new day and brand new things happen and it's true for our patients and some of those things, those new things that happen, can be incredibly overwhelming, particularly when people are coming to the end of life. And somehow just to be there alongside them and being on that journey of discovery with them I think is a way of giving spiritual care. So just being able to listen, listen beyond words, listen to what's really coming from somewhere deeper and trying to learn that intuitive ability of actually not just hearing someone's words…but actually there is maybe something much deeper behind those words…and not necessarily coming to conclusions about that but just being aware of that…and listening in case that person wants to talk through that (participant 8)

He goes on to propose that the ability to connect with something deeper in people can be learned, and that once 'felt', the power of this investment in another becomes almost addictive, and potentially perpetuates an ability to focus on spirituality:

> I think you can learn to do it. I think some people are naturally more able to do that, just partly their personality or their life experiences that brought them to that point. But I think once you've done it once or twice, once you've actually tried to connect with something deeper in people once or twice, and you see how powerful that is, you get hooked in! And you keep on doing it and it keeps on happening and it reinforces continuously that whole spirituality thing really (participant 8)

However, apart from personality and life experience, an individual's aptitude to learn this skill is seen to be dependent on their approach to patient care. Fredriksson[8] describes two modes of relating to caring conversation. One mode is that of contact in which nurses 'hear' what the patient needs, completes the necessary task, and so their presence in 'being there' for patients is one of problem solving. This mode appears to equate with the 'very efficient' nurse, described below, who may have difficulty in connecting with something deeper in others. Fredricksson's[9] second mode is one of connection in which nurses 'listen', and so not only remain silent them- selves but also silence their mind so that it is not distracted by other thoughts. Therefore they focus on 'being with' the patient they are caring for at that moment:

It also depends where people have come from, where they've worked, their working background, so you've got some staff who are very efficient and need to get the tasks done, and the task is the focus, and then you've got other staff that actually the task is secondary and the core of a person is much more important, and trying to connect with that. And of course you can't forget the tasks, and that's the difficult thing isn't it, it's trying to find that balance really. Because it's very easy to just suddenly forget about the tasks completely, which is very impractical, I mean spirituality is earthy at the end of the day so actually giving someone a wash is spiritual (participant 8)

One of the youngest participants not only emphasized the value of listening to patients, but also evidenced her awareness of the implications of age difference on understanding feelings. However, this does not detract from her using the present moment of nurse–patient interface to encourage coping, by sharing her positive observations of aspects of the patient's current situation:

To be able to listen to someone, and obviously for me I'm very young and you don't want to patronize them if they're very old, that's…you know, I don't think that's appropriate, what do I know? I'm not that age, I couldn't possibly understand what they're feeling, but I can listen. I can…maybe point out things that are happening in their life that is good, that are going well, or family that is supportive, or things that they are doing, to maybe show that there are some things that are good in life (participant 11)

TIME AS A COMMODITY

Time as a commodity was inferred, or referred to, by many respondents in their accounts of communicating and being with patients. It was important that patients had 'got' time to talk to the nurse, and for the nurse, time provided the means of building relationships with patients:

To be with people so they've got time to actually tell you what their need is or even just to sit with them so they can talk generally so you've got more to build on the basic relationship (participant 5)

One participant's experience reflected the need for patience in 'giving' time to those in her care. Patient and relative stories that were reiterated over and over again were seen as being potentially beneficial for them, and therefore the nurse felt it her duty to give the time to listen to their story each time it was recounted:

…they have experienced a tremendous amount along the way to the point where we see them when they come in. I think it is really important, that we…remember that and give and enable the patient and relatives to retrace their steps sometimes and we see it often, some families don't want to go there, but others have to go there time and time again, they have to retrace their steps and they have to verbalize their journey over and over again. And sometimes it's hard, you think, oh I've heard all this before, but I think you need to stop and think no, I've got to give them this time to get there because I feel they're beginning their healing process by doing that if that's what they need to do (participant 2)

Another participant appeared responsive in 'finding' time for unplanned, but significant conversation that 'always' commenced at the moment of leaving a patient's home. The skill is described as not trying to answer the unanswerable, but as letting the 'other', whether they be patient or relative, just bounce their concerns off you:

…and there's always the door, as you're going out of the door, the question – always happen don't they – you know, the husband will say how long is it going to be, or what's it going to be like? And then you get into the whole conversation bit, you know, you can be stood on the doorstep for half an hour. And it's realizing that 'gosh, that's where the work's done'…I think the real skills have come in dealing with those questions that can't be answered, but just giving time really, just letting them just bounce off you I suppose (participant 9)

Being sensitive to communication needs in this way is both compassionate and authentic.[10] The physical presence of nurses as professional carers 'being there' for patients and relatives is moved on to their 'being with' them psychologically.[11]

CLOSED SITUATIONS

Sometimes, despite attempts to develop a trusting relationship, patients were unable or unwilling to share what was troubling them:

We had somebody once who…the problem was she didn't…you couldn't get to the bottom of her pain and sometimes she would start to talk about other things that were obviously on her mind, but if you tried to follow that through suddenly she would be in terrible pain and you would have to go and get something for the pain and you'd think actually a lot of the pain is spiritual pain and she started to deal with it and then couldn't, couldn't deal with it. It seemed very much [that] way anyway…She was in so much pain in the end but still no…and should have been totally sedated really, it seemed like she was but she was very well aware of things still and I remember going to talk to her and just gently touched her hand and then said something to her and you'd have thought she barely wasn't conscious and she said 'oh that's…whoever you are, I know the arms, I know who you are' so she was very well aware still of what was going on. And still very agitated, but she just wouldn't open up about it. I mean we had half an idea about some things but it never all came out. She just wouldn't deal with it (participant 7)

If talking through situations is a primary source of support in helping patients and relatives cope by 'processing', or making sense of their situation, how do professionals support those who do not want to know the details?

You know, you can only be there to try and support them and talk them through things that have happened, why they've happened, how they've happened, what then happened…you know what I mean, you know, if an event happened, explaining to them, well this happened for these reasons and because of these reasons it's like a spiral… just trying to let them be able to process the actual situation. Because it's so tragic that sometimes you just need…I think the facts help…But then you do get people who don't want to know anything and then that's very difficult because…especially if, say, for example, somebody's diagnosed with cancer – they don't want to know…how do you support somebody who doesn't want to know what you know about them, how can you support them as a whole person through their journey if they can't accept it themselves? (participant 12)

The answer to the question posed, at least in part, appears in participant 12's own description in 'being there', and in her action in respecting their decision not to talk about it until they are ready do so

REPLENISHMENT

Nurses need to maintain their own well-being, their personal spiritual integrity, if they are to provide spiritual care in situations of loss. Therefore the nurse's commitment to companion-ship in her professional caring role needs to be offset by a life outside the work environment that has its own richness so that relationships with patients remain balanced.[12] A number of respondents describe ways in which they get back to 'being themselves' outside of the work environment. The first interviewee found it quite difficult to find the right words to describe the need for some sort of recovery from a 'bad' day at work or a feeling that is not quite feel-ing 'down'. She eventually described needing replenishment, a term that could apply to other participants' experience:

If I've had a bad day at work, Locatelli's violin concertos cheer me up no end. No it's not cheering me up, it's sort of…I wouldn't say I go home feeling down because that's not the right expression, but sort of listening to that music it just does something for me…Looking at art, it certainly absolutely lifts my spirit, a very big thing. That has always been the case, although I've never really thought about it much…and to a slightly lesser degree being at home and doing something I like to do. So if I had no time for that then I would feel that I would not be sort of replenished (participant 1)

The means of getting back to being themselves, for some, seemed to be associated with solitary activities. Participant 8 makes regular, formal arrangements to be alone in order to find space to reconnect with himself:

I'll go away for a weekend in retreat…where I am just on my own and just find the space to be myself and not to have to think about anything particularly but just to go for long walks or just be in my own company and I might sit in silence, look at the view, just try and reconnect with myself, get in touch with myself again a little bit. Because quite often when you're just dealing with people, tasks and things you feel as if you're part of a process, you aren't actually really feeling in touch with yourself, not feeling grounded in yourself. And I find that (at retreat) I can bring myself back into myself… (participant 8)

Similarly, participant 12 chooses to spend time out without human company to lift her mood, perhaps providing a break from any expectation to communicate:

I garden! I have a greenhouse so I potter around in there for a while, and I walk the dogs, so they're my two things really (participant 12)

Key for several other participants is the balance that home life offers:

…I do believe home has got to be…your outside of work life has got to be in good balance for you to be able to work here effectively (participant 2)

Family responsibilities appeared to be an effective distraction from work. The contrast in environment and activities shifted perspective, for example:

For me personally though it's also having a family so you're not doing that all day every day, you go home and do something completely different (participant 6)

One respondent implied that the journey home allowed for the transition from the role of the nurse to a return to being a mum again:

I tend to find, to be honest, that by the time I get home, you walk in the door and you become a mum again, you haven't time actually to be thinking about work too much and dealing with all the problems that are thrown at you the minute you walk in the door. I think it is important as well to have a life outside, to have things that you're busy with… Because otherwise it probably would be easy to take it [work] home (participant 7)

Another respondent seemed to have a more complex home life with her family commitments often being 'elsewhere' and so outside the home after work:

But I think on a daily basis you do have to get on, you know, I've got a family at home and, nine times out of ten, I've commitments elsewhere so I have to meet those commitments regardless of what's happened at work (participant 5)

In the same way that participants have identified that listening to patients and giving them time to talk through their concerns is important, so too many of these participants turn to their wife, husband, boyfriend or parents at home for a listening ear to talk through their concerns. Some identified what their chosen confidant had to offer, for example participant 8 valued his wife's understanding, but also her being a nurse was mentioned, and therefore probably significant:

I mean I talk to my wife…she's a nurse…she's very understanding so I can talk to her about anything, anything goes (participant 8)

Participant 12 was explicit in valuing her parents nursing experience in using them as a support network:

…both my parents are nurses so I have my own little sort of support network and they've obviously been through other experiences, so I can always chat to them about my thoughts and feelings and things (participant 12)

The implication from participant 10 is that support at home is more their ability to accommodate the emotional state in which she arrives after work:

Sometimes I'll go home and talk to my husband, but I think sometimes I go home and am quiet, or I'm angry with everybody (participant 10)

Humour can be used to protect, to maintain an appropriate distance.[13] Participant 8 made a collective claim that 'loads of people' in palliative care rely on a sense of humour to maintain a balanced perspective. He explains how he works at fuelling his humour at home with friends as a means of completely 'being' himself:

But I think one thing that's massively important, and I think loads of people would tell you this in palliative care, is to have a sense of humour…If you haven't got a sense of humour you're doomed…I try and watch comedies as much as I can, and have a really good laugh, because I think that just releases so many good chemicals and they're so good for you. And to be with friends who you can just be completely yourself with, be the biggest fool, and just have a really good laugh, a real belly laugh (participant 8)

His claim is supported by respondent 10, who after describing palliative patient scenarios she had experienced, believed that to survive it was important to partake in activities to lighten mood:

I try and do something light-hearted, watch some silly television programme or read a book, but nothing…something quite light-hearted really, trying to change my mood. That's what I tend to do. If I want to read a book or watch TV it's got to have a happy ending! (participant 10)

SUMMARY

In choosing how we are with, and how we treat, others we reflect our potential for being spiritual; in nursing it is conveyed in the way care is provided. Establishing a rapport with patients is fundamental to identifying their needs. Communication that reflects spiritual care is 'connected'. It is patient-focused, and triggered by the emotional insight of the carer, which enables them to identify with the sufferer. Caring conversation is generally the preferred means of participants' exploring the patient's spiritual needs. However, one participant felt a written document, including guiding questions, was useful in initiating a spiritual assessment. Verbal communication was not always considered necessary in establishing a rapport, but the supportive presence of just sitting with a patient could induce sufficient confidence to enable them to begin to share their worst fears. The process of active listening facilitates the listener's potential in reaching for meaning to gain a deeper understanding of need and so contributes to a better interpretation of what is being said. Active listening is a means of sharing oneself, and can both facilitate identifying spiritual need and be a source of spiritual care. This was evident in participant comments that suggest the need to 'give' or 'find' time to ensure patients had time to 'talk'. Metaphor was used by several nurses to share 'a sense of' the experience they were trying to convey. Participants' own spiritual well-being is maintained in various ways, through solitary activities, the distraction of home life, a friend or relative's 'listening ear' and a sense of humour to maintain a balanced perspective.

REFERENCES

1. Morse JM, Bottorff J, Anderson G *et al.* Beyond empathy: expanding expressions of caring. *Journal of Advanced Nursing.* 1992; **17**: 809–21.
2. James N. Emotional labour: skill and work in social regulation of feelings. *Sociological Review.* 1989; **37**(1): 15–42.
3. Fredriksson L. The caring conversation – talking about suffering: a hermeneutic phenomenological studying psychiatric nursing. *International Journal for Human Caring.* 1998; **1**: 24–32.
4. Ewles L and Simnett I. *Promoting Health: a Practical Guide.* Edinburgh: Bailliere Tindall, 2003.
5. McLeod DL and Wright LM. Living the as-yet unanswered: spiritual care practices in family systems nursing. *Journal of Family Nursing.* 2008; **14**(1): 118–41.

6. Pettigrew J. Intensive nursing care-the ministry of presence. *Critical Care Nursing Clinics of North America*. 1990; **3**: 503–8.

7. Kemper BJ. Therapeutic listening: developing the concept. *Journal of Psychosocial Nursing and Mental Health Services*. 1992; **7**: 21–3.

8. Fredriksson L. Modes of relating in caring conversation: a research synthesis on presence, touch and listening. *Journal of Advanced Nursing*. 1999; **30**(5): 1167–76.

9. Ibid.

10. Golberg B. Connection: an exploration of spirituality in nursing care. *Journal of Advanced Nursing*. 1998; **27**(4): 836–42.

11. Speck P, Higginson I and Addington-Hall J. Spiritual needs in healthcare. *BMJ*. 2004; **329**: 123–4.

12. Campbell A. *Moderated Love: A Theology of Professional Care*. London: SPCK, 1984.

13. Davies B and Oberle K. Dimensions of the supportive role of the nurse in palliative care. *Oncology Nursing Forum*. 1990; **17**(1): 87–94.

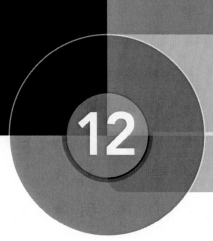

Becoming proficient in spiritual care

12

Adulthood in western society is associated with a sense of control.[1] Generations grow and are educated in a culture that values individualism, technological and scientific advancement. Such advancement provides an increasing expectation of individual choice. Research participants' experience provided examples of how spiritual care was individualized, and how patients and their relatives were enabled to make real choices that were meaningful and facilitated coping. Nurses' accounts of personal loss were powerful in conveying how they had grown in the face of suffering, and how this had empowered them in practice situations involving loss.

FACILITATION OF RELIGIOUS PRACTICE AS A SPIRITUAL RESOURCE

Where religious practice was a component of patient spirituality, individualising patient access to religious ritual or service facilitated a potential means of coping. This was achieved by participants' negotiating and organizing skills, so patients' needs were attended to as appropriate; for example, in community practice:

…making sure that all of the things with regards to her religion and her well-being, because you know that's what she believes in and making sure that we could do all those things, getting priests, and you know, making sure that she could have communion at home and all those sorts of things (participant 12)

…and in the nursing home:

We have the local Church of England and a Baptist church come here and they do like a monthly service, so there's a service every two weeks. And then there's a few people, three from downstairs and two from upstairs, who go locally to the service on Sunday, a Roman Catholic service (participant 3)

Nurses differentiate between their personal beliefs and those of their patient:

> I think you still keep your own beliefs and spirituality, just because they don't (share these particular beliefs) it doesn't affect how that patient is nursed and you certainly would not enforce your own particular beliefs on the patient (participant 9)

Most nurses who are religious themselves are aware that their faith affects their outlook, and so, almost self-consciously, were looking for 'the other's' perspective on faith so their own views did not get in the way, for example:

> Spirituality to me is about my religion…I think that probably colours my outlook a little bit. But I know lots of people don't have religion or are not bothered by it, so I think you have to be aware that other people see things differently. And you have to go by them more and their outlook on things when you're looking after people, you can't impose yours, your beliefs and outlooks onto someone else (participant 10)

However, one participant described how she did not 'inflict' her religious beliefs on others, but throughout her interview she did tend to 'talk' in religious terms. She seemed to lack any awareness of this tendency when she goes on to describe how she found that patients tended to 'pick up' on her religious faith, and that this facilitated conversation about religion:

> I'm a practising Christian but I'll never inflict my views on anybody else although very often they'll pick up on it and therefore it is a topic of conversation and that really is quite helpful when you're dealing with people who are dying (participant 4)

The importance of not proselytizing was so important to one participant that she implied that she did not address religion at all when caring for patients. Such a restricted view may well limit this nurse's ability to facilitate fulfilment of patients' religion-based spiritual needs:

> Because I certainly wouldn't give any religious input to anybody, that's…as an individual… so I would never…that's not something for me to talk about (participant 11)

In reality, given the space to do so, the patient often leads in making requests for religious activities that help them cope:

> I think your path's set out for you by the patient, I think they lead, they'll lead the way. You might be asking the right questions at the right time, but I think they'll lead the way. They'll let you know…I was just thinking of a past [patient] that I've had, [who had] a very

strong belief, and yes she drove where she wanted to go and where she wanted to be and how she wanted to incorporate her spirituality into her dying (participant 9)

Some requests involved nurses in religious ritual. One participant was asked to pray for a patient, and was both pleased with, and emotionally moved by, the outcome:

And anyway we started building up like a working relationship from then, and one time I went in there and she said...she asked me if I prayed and I said 'yes I do pray every night' and she asked me to pray for her. And so I sat and it's the first time I've ever prayed with somebody...and I said this prayer and it came out really good. And she was having a cry afterwards, I was having a cry afterwards, and I don't know...she just seemed more relaxed after that (participant 3)

A hospice nurse explains how she has been asked both to read the Bible and to pray with patients. It is not difficult to envisage the comfort such activities may offer, not only in hearing the words spoken but also in possibly bringing some familiarity of worship where others read the Bible and prayers are said together:

Well, there have been patients who've asked me to read from the Bible for them...Or when people ask you to pray with them, I mean it does happen sometimes (participant 1)

Patient requests can surprise nurses. A community nurse thought it 'strange' when a patient she had known for years, who had not appeared to be practising a religious faith, asked her to get his Bible from a cupboard. The Bible was a school Bible, which evidenced his early grounding in Christian faith. He was also specific in the text he wanted to read, which further suggested that that grounding was thorough, or that he had in some way maintained his biblical knowledge throughout his life. The nurse also thought it 'strange' that he wanted to read from the book of Job, which she described as 'very dark and questioning':

But towards the end, I suppose about three or four weeks maybe, really quite [near] to the end, [he] was insistent that the Bible was at the bedside and I'd never seen his Bible before but [it] was brought out of the cupboard and it was [an] old Bible from school... and he picked it up and read Job, you know, it seems awful but to me it's very dark and questioning (participant 9)

She continued to reflect on his background, appearing to be trying to make sense of this situation herself, and recalled that his background might 'shed a little light' on that because, that was also 'strange'. Born in India, he had been pressured into religion as a child and had since, at least in part, rejected that religion to make up his own mind:

I'd known the gentleman for some time, years in fact, and you know, nursed him through that coping, that acceptance of what he was going to reach and face, it was really quite bizarre. And quite young as well, so…hmm. But the background was really quite strange, it might just shed a little light on that, which is probably where it came to, was his parents were missionaries in India and he was born in India and lived in India and had said at one point that he had the belief but he felt pressurized as a child and lost part of his religion because it was enforced on him, I think maybe he felt he needed to make his own mind up. So [he] wasn't actually practising as far as I knew…had just brought it up on initial assessment and then that was gone…for a couple of years… (participant 9)

In the same way as most of the participants were introduced to religion in their childhood and moved away from overt practice in their youth, only for some to later rediscover their faith, it is not unreasonable to consider that some patients may have done exactly the same, particularly in the light of Culliford's[2] consideration of this phenomenon (see Chapter 10). Also, this man was dying and may well have felt that his situation was dark, and one which might well engender questioning. Bible stories often reflect life situations and can offer hope for those who have faith. Job's faith saw him through difficulty so that his 'latter days were more than his beginning'.[3] Hence, although perhaps not understanding her patient's choice, in complying with his request she may well have facilitated his coping.

In other ways, nurses lead in the identification and means of fulfilling patients' needs of religious practice. One participant 'checked out' the boundaries of her personal ability to meet a patient's need by looking to the Chaplain for support:

And sometimes people do actually ask you things sort of about God or relating to – I talk about Christian religion here [it] is the only thing I experience here at work – and people might ask questions which are about the existence of God…once somebody had read this chapter from the Bible and I felt I was able to answer but also sort of went to the Chaplain…I just think that surely he's far better than I am obviously to deal with that, and possibly probe further if that is the right word (participant 1)

Another respondent intentionally raised the issue of religious practice when in conversation with residents on their admission to the nursing home. Her rationale for being so direct in enquiry regarding religious needs was that she anticipated that many residents may have a view on religious practice due to their generation:

…and I talk to them and say you know are you a church goer, do you have contact with the church, and a lot of them do because a lot of them are of the generation where they've spent their lives in a church scenario. Once they come in here that makes it very difficult… so I go through with them what it means coming here and what can I do to help, and I'll often arrange whatever they want to come and visit them. If they have no church but they'd like to see a minister we usually get the chap in from Age…you know, the Church of England, if it's Baptist I'll get a Baptist minister. You know, I will always try and find somebody appropriate (participant 4)

EMPOWERMENT OF PATIENTS

Hope is an integral part of spirituality, and is a powerful coping mechanism in times of duress. A dominant component of hope is the personal dimension or spirit of hope, which involves meaning associated with a sense of the possible or a feeling of empowerment.[4] Any sense of loss of value potentially challenges hope. Hence individuals whose health is declining or who are informed of the terminal nature of their condition can feel 'written off' or valueless and loose hope.[5] This is exacerbated as the need to relinquish significant roles related to 'who they were' is increasingly associated with dependence on others. Respondents' accounts of their experiences include several examples of this. Each respondent's example differed, as did the means of helping patients. However, they all reflected a fundamental understanding of the value of facilitating patient empowerment by giving or allowing them real choice and thus some control over the measures they could take in coping with their situation.

One example reflects how liberating choosing to join the hospice's creative writing group was for a particular patient and their relative. Writing not only helped them express themselves, but also helped them face and deal with their issues. Certainly the therapeutic benefits of writing are reported as a way of making sense of loss associated with dying.[6]

> …they have art group here in day therapy…and…creative writing groups…I remember with the first creative writing group…this book was produced…and I have actually spoken to a patient and husband of a patient who joined that, and say how positive it was…how it helped them [in]…expressing and therefore facing and dealing with certain issues… and…the art group…people do find it positive actually making or creating art themselves (participant 1)

Similarly, art provides a way of exploring the deeper meaning of being, of understanding existential issues related to dying that are not easily expressed in words.[7] It is well established as a therapeutic tool that can gradually awaken or illuminate patient perceptions in situations of loss.[8,9]

> …they say that by being involved in something like that it takes their mind off things completely, which I suppose is very important, I suppose an incurable illness is something that weighs on your mind all the time, so they do say 'it really takes my mind off something', and then 'being able to share it with others' is something that is said. I like to think there may be something a bit deeper as well that they can't explain in words, or I can't put in words! (participant 1)

Another scenario concerned a young women who was dying and found it difficult coming to terms with the loss of her role as a mother. She repeatedly expressed her feelings of complete failure in not being able to take care of her boys. However, she was encouraged to create memory boxes for her sons, which would help them remember their relationship with her after her death.[10] On the occasions she was well enough to return home for a day, she was able to pick up items of her own choosing for this endeavour. In this small way she was still able to 'do' something for her boys, and the nursing staff felt this helped her come to terms with her situation:

> I'm thinking of a young mother and two boys. And the loss of her role as a mum…it affected her tremendously. She used to talk about it to us and various members of staff, whoever was with her really, caring for her. She just used to talk about how she couldn't do these things for the boys any longer and she just felt a complete failure. And it hurt…I think it probably hurt her more than anything…I think putting together memory boxes for her boys helped her come to terms with that, because she was once again doing something for them…I don't think she ever completed them but…she went home on day leave from here more than once and I think when she was home she picked up things from the house and put them in these memory boxes for the boys. And we felt that compensated a little for the losses she was feeling about not being able to do anything for them (participant 2)

A further example was a woman who had been beautiful, and who struggled to deal with the change in her appearance, that was due to the side effects of the medication she took to manage her illness. She also had a young son who drew a picture of how he saw his 'mum'. This drawing provided her with an alternative perspective in reminding her of the 'self' that was not lost, her enduring role as a mother. She used this drawing as a source of coping by choosing to cover her mirror with it, and in this way had a more positive view of her 'self':

> …I remember a lady here…she was, you know, stunningly beautiful before she was ill and took loads of steroids [due to] the illness, and from when she was admitted the first time to when she was admitted the second time you wouldn't have recognized her, nobody would have recognized her. And for her…well for anyone, but particularly because of the type of person she was, that was hugely difficult to deal with, so she couldn't look in the mirror, because she'd lost the person that she was, she wouldn't look in the mirror. So her little boy drew a picture of her and how he saw her and she stuck that on the mirror so that when she looked at it, that's what she saw was how he saw her, not what she looked like now (participant 6)

These examples have all been taken from the experience of nurses working in a hospice environment. The hospice in question benefits from a number of resources that include the provision of therapies such as art and creative writing. They also include a family support service that would have been available to help both the children and parents involved in the latter two scenarios. The availability of these resources clearly facilitated the hospice nurses' empowerment of their patients.

Patient empowerment was also exemplified by the experiences of some nurses in the community and nursing home environments. This was primarily by advocating for patients' interest,[11] which was necessary when the choices patients had made in coping with their own death were challenged by their relatives. One example of this concerned a matter of ensuring that a patient's decision of 'how' she wanted to die was respected. The participant, a community nurse, explained that one patient, who was a nurse herself, knew that she was dying and was very prepared and organized in what she wanted. Her decisions were based on her strong religious faith and her professional understanding of medication for management of her symptoms. However, her husband, a consultant who primarily dealt with medical emergencies, wanted her life to be prolonged and pressed for more active medical intervention. The community nurse showed an understanding of the consultant's 'mindset':

And she had a very strong faith herself, a strong Catholic faith, she knew she was dying. She had everything prepared, she had organized everything, we did what she wanted, she had the drugs that she felt she needed, she had the care she felt she needed, but it was quite hard on a couple of occasions. One particular occasion when her husband cornered me in the kitchen because I was getting her syringe driver drugs...I think looking after somebody in their terminal stages takes [a] different mindset to an...consultant, because we know we're not going to make somebody better, our aim is to provide somebody with a good death. The death that they wanted, as pain-free as possible, and in a way that they wanted, and acknowledging the fact that that's going to happen. Whereas as an... consultant, it was also his wife so he obviously loved her dearly, [he] does not normally look after somebody who's dying, their aim is to...get them well and send them on their way, so he was trying to make suggestions about what we should do with her drugs to make her better (participant 10)

The organizational structure of nursing services is hierarchical, whereas doctors work in collegiate systems. Consequently, nurses may be caught in divided loyalties between patient and doctor.[12] Although 'outranked' in professional kudos by the consultant, the nurse remained adamant in her responsibility for her patient, and explained why she needed to respect her patient's choice of care, as she would, presumably, to any husband.

...[I] explained to him as best I could that if we changed the drugs to what he wanted it wouldn't alter the outcome and to remind him that was not what she wanted and we had to do what she wanted because she was our patient, and she was the main reason we were there and what she wanted was what we had to do. And that we understood that he felt hopeless and he didn't want to lose her, but perhaps he should spend some more time talking to her (participant 10)

This same participant gave another example of how a patient's choice of 'when' she would die was respected. The patient appeared to have decided that she had had enough and wanted to die sooner rather than later. She said she could not eat because of nausea and retching, but she had never been seen to retch by anyone, and so perhaps not surprisingly, measures to assuage theses symptoms were ineffective. Her family was frustrated by the patient's apparent determination not to eat:

She'd decided that she'd had enough and wanted to die, but she hadn't quite reached the end stage of her life...but she was almost forcing herself to. So she was ready but her family weren't. They were finding it hard. So you had her saying that she couldn't eat, and that she's feeling nauseous all the time. And the family are saying she is eating, there's nothing wrong. And that caused a bit of a…sort of tug between the family and the patient for us nurses, because the family were saying they want one thing and then the patient says she wants another. So you have to go with the patient, it's their decision…with this particular lady we'd tried every single drug we can find to stop her feeling all this nausea and this retching but nothing seems to be working but nobody actually saw her retch at all, but she said she was doing it all the time. So I think it was her way of saying I've had enough, I don't want to eat or drink anymore, I just want to go now (participant 10)

Patients may understand self-empowerment by choosing to shorten the period they live with dying by not eating, and so hasten death. The nurse rightly understands that she needs to advocate for the patient's right to choose in a situation where the family are confrontational. However, she was also right to feel uneasy when the patient requests opioid analgesia without any apparent symptoms of suffering pain. There is a significant ethical difference between a competent patient's right to decline healthcare offered[13] and the nurse being asked to administer medication to hasten death:

…she told us that she was in pain and the dilemma was – I wasn't convinced she was in pain, I think she was just asking for diamorphine because she thought it might speed things along. But the dilemma is she told us she was in pain. Somebody's perception of pain is what they tell you…She was just a determined lady who'd made her mind up. And so she was going to take herself to bed and die (participant 10)

Friction in families was also experienced in the nursing home environment. On this occasion, rather than a particular patient scenario, the participant makes a general comment about the pattern of families appearing in relation to the timing of patients dying. Accepted practice allows competent patients to make their wishes regarding future treatment known by written statement or witnessed oral statements.[14] Participant 5 sees the increased tendency for people to write down what they want as the 'means' of empowering dying residents. The implication is that by formally recording their choices while they are still well enough to speak for themselves, the dying will not be overwhelmed by their families' wishes as they weaken:

Friction between families is something that is difficult at times, you know, we have people that have been here for years, never had a visitor, then in the last days of their life there is a descent of people that you've never met before suddenly are here…It is very difficult. I think now…with more people writing out their last wills…I think residents' choice, you know it will be easier for them to write down what they want before maybe it gets to that stage…I think maybe the family have to see that paper, [identifying the patient's wishes]… it maybe would make them think…I don't think they realize how overwhelming they're being at times (participant 5)

EMPOWERMENT OF SUPPORT STAFF

In the nursing home environment the needs of individuals vary, with some only needing supportive care. Consequently, one or two registered nurses manage a team of care assistants/support workers on each 'floor' of the nursing home. The registered nurses were aware of the need to promote, and maintain, awareness of whole person care, particularly among the young inexperienced support workers:

…and we have a really, really good team. And it's about the strong helping the weak. And it's very difficult, some of them are very young and you have to be really careful that looking after clients doesn't become just a routine, you know, you wash and feed and change them, wash and feed and change them, get them up, put them back to bed, wash and change them…you know, and it can become very rote (participant 4)

The implication is that those made strong by knowledge or experience help those who are 'weak' in either or both. In this way, the experienced can empower the novice carer to understand the importance of holistic care as the bedrock of facilitating coping.

Another nursing home respondent describes the range of skills found amongst the support staff as being very mixed. Relevant experience in end of life care is conveyed as being rather random, through personal life or past working experience. She also implies a similar awareness to that of participant 4 above, in that some support staff consider their role as one of tasks to complete rather than having a more vocational view of caring, described below as the 'bigger picture':

I think we've got such a wide skill mix, we've got very young girls to staff of retirement age. Some have had prior experience in care homes, some haven't. Some have had a lot of things happen through their own personal lives, whereas obviously youngsters maybe wouldn't have been through so much that they can relate to. And it's how they view their job role, I think some of them believe that, you know, they look at their job description in black and white, they feel they're coming in to wash people, dress people, feed people. Not all of them see the bigger picture. I'm not saying that's through their fault but that's through their training or their understanding of the role when they take it on (participant 5)

This participant goes on to acknowledge the culture shock, and potential fear, for inexperienced support workers in dealing with death, and compares this with the inevitable preparation that all registered nurses have to undergo regarding caring for dying patients. She implies some hope for 'change' as training may empower all support workers to contribute more effectively in the care of the dying. The Liverpool Care Pathway that she refers to is a protocol for addressing the last days of a patient's life.[15] This guidance reflects holistic hospice philosophy in attending to essential physical, psychological and spiritual needs of the dying person as well as the communication and bereavement needs of their significant others.

I mean they are doing the Liverpool Care [Pathway] as part of their training now here, they've started doing it, so perhaps it will start to change, but there is a huge difference in skills. Whereas as a nurse, when you train to be a nurse, you can't avoid death, you know yourself you have to go…you're going to look after people that die, you're going to be with those relatives and you're going to be involved in that situation and a carer, [they've not] necessarily…had any prior training so they wouldn't have been. So some of them I think maybe haven't thought it through and realized that or they are really frightened of it themselves and they keep away (participant 5)

One nursing home participant described how she had overheard well-meaning support workers offer patients empty reassurance:

…they're really worried about something and the carer just tells them 'Oh well it'll be fine, they'll sort it out'. And you know full well they won't sort it out, because you know what the problem is, and so the person might feel that they can't discuss it, they might feel they can't. You know what I mean, you think…are they trying to sort of shut them up or are they just trying to make themselves feel better? (participant 3)

She had set up a spiritual reflection group in her workplace that was aimed primarily, but not exclusively, at support staff. Attendance at this group was voluntary. In helping those who attended the sessions develop an understanding of what is meant by the term 'spirituality' and increase their awareness of how this relates to their work, this practitioner empowers them to choose how they think about and approach caring for residents. In this way support workers are potentially better able to assist residents and registered nurses in their facilitation of residents' coping strategies.

I've started addressing these sort of issues in…things like the spiritual care support reflection groups which normally get between six and eight staff at a time…I tend to do like two sessions, I do like a first one where we just talk about what spirituality is and how it is relevant to our work and look at examples which I've taken from literature. And sometimes in that first session they'll start relating it to their own work, and sometimes they won't, it depends on the group you've got. And then the second group, I do this sort of like reflection of issues to do [with] their work so they have to start thinking and bringing up things and thinking along the lines of…how right was it, how wrong was it, could it have been done differently, and all that sort of thing (participant 3)

PERSONAL LOSS AS A SOURCE OF ENHANCED UNDERSTANDING AND POSITIVE GROWTH

Some nurses' personal stories reflect what Bury[16] refers to as biographical disruption, where illness or a particular traumatic event appears to have led to a re-examination of life issues in relation to the diagnosis of disease or the incident in question.

Participant 9, for example, described how her personal experience of loss had made her aware of how little she had really understood previously about the process of grief. She reflects on how, despite her interest in psychology, and her understanding of grief theory, she had no real depth of understanding of what the phases, stages or words used to describe the process of grief meant until she lost her father. The impact of personal loss on professional perspective has been described by others.[17] In this instance the nurse's professional understanding appears enriched by her personal experience:

I think…until I lost my father I don't think I fully understood what loss and bereavement was, felt like. I've always been kind of interested in psychology if you like, and have read quite a bit on loss and bereavement. I think we were all brought up…with Kubler-Ross with her seven stages,…and I hope I remember the seven stages and going down them and thinking yes that's the reaction that she talks about, and yes that's perfectly understandable and people work that way, but until I lost my father I think I don't really…I didn't fully understand what those phases were, when she talks about guilt and bargaining and anger and denial and all of those things, I think they were just words that you could pick out in a dictionary and look to see what the meaning was, but until you've actually experienced it yourself…I don't think I had any depth to my knowledge other than having read research papers or books on loss and bereavement or attended hospice lectures and that sort of thing. So I think for me, I very much had to experience it and it was quite late in life,…because I didn't really know my grandparents and was lucky enough not to have lost anybody near and dear until I was sort of 50 really. Well, mid-40s. So it's personal experience of loss that gave me depth to maybe some of the knowledge that I had (participant 9)

Similarly, participant 2 describes how her personal encounter with grief following the loss of her son partly accounts for her taking a nursing post in a hospice. She uses metaphor to describe the impact of her son's suicide, and tries to make sense of the situation in asking 'why':

And that threw my world just up in the air and it came crashing down in bits and pieces… from thinking that I couldn't go on and why had this happened to me, to us as a family, I – from that very dark place – with the support of both family and friends, and I have to say my faith, and my attitude to life that you can't be in control of other people…And at the time I asked all these questions: Why? What have I done wrong? I wasn't a good enough mother? 9½ years later I'm strong again, and during…about six months after James died I sort of decided that I had to get on with my life and what was I going to do with it, I didn't want to retire, I wanted to carry on nursing, and that's when I saw an advert for a post at the…hospice as a staff nurse. And when the hospice opened I thought, oh I'd like to work there, and I felt this was my opportunity. Because I had (a) close bereavement I was advised not to start until 12 months after my bereavement and in fact I started there 10 months after my bereavement (participant 2)

This participant's experience illustrates how the emotional response to loss, such as anger, although potentially destructive, can also energize individuals into positive activities that are a direct result of the loss.[18] She has, for example, come to regard the tragedy of the loss of her son as one of growth, in that it has opened opportunities that have enriched her life and professional practice, for example she feels able to offer support through a national support line to others bereaved by suicide.

Also, she feels she is able to be more empathetic towards patients and their families who have had to cope with loss and bereavement. In an interpretative phenomenological study focused on the experience of nine older adult Christians' search for meaning following the loss of their partners, Golsworthy and Coyle[19] also found that participants spoke of an enhanced capacity for empathy and understanding of others.

In addition, knowing that three people have benefited from the donation of her son's organs has helped this participant make sense of personal tragedy:

And my experience with losing my son really gave me a lot of empathy towards the families, the patients and families I was looking after. And spiritually I felt that this is one good thing that has come out of losing a son – which one would never ever want to. And other good things have happened as a result of losing James which have enriched my life. One of those being…we were able to donate some of his organs when he died and three people have got new life because of the loss of his life, which I'm eternally grateful for, because it has given me a very positive aspect to my bereavement and my grief. And latterly, the last three years, I've been supporting other people who have or are trying to survive a bereavement by suicide, by manning a national support helpline – the acronym is SOBS – it's Survivors of Bereavement by Suicide (participant 2)

The same respondent describes how life experience helps the development and growth of the spiritual self as a source of strength and a resource which better enables us to support others:

I think spirituality develops within a person as that person grows in age and life experience. I think it changes through life and life's experience…it's how we see life and how we get through life's challenges, whether they're good or not so good. It's our strength, which enables us to cope with different situations. And also it's a strength that helps us help other people, because of our own life experience and how those experiences have helped us develop our spirituality (participant 2)

SUMMARY

Where religious practice was a component of patient spirituality nurses endeavoured to individualize patient access to religious ritual or service. Hope is an integral part of spirituality, and involves meaning associated with a sense of the possible or a feeling of empowerment. In facilitating patient empowerment or advocating for their right to make choices, participants provided patients with a measure of control in coping with situations of loss. Examples included art as a means of understanding existential issues that are not easily expressed in words, and the encouragement of a mother to create memory boxes for her sons which would help them remember their relationship with her. Advocacy was necessary when the choices patients had made in coping with their own death were challenged by their relatives. Inexperienced support workers also needed to be empowered to cope with the culture shock and fear of dealing with death, as well as to understand that empty reassurance is inappropriate in these situations. The experience of personal loss appears particularly powerful in strengthening nurses' empathy for patients who are struggling to 'make sense of' and cope with loss.

REFERENCES

1. Friedemann M, Mouch J and Racey T. Nursing the spirit: the framework of systemic organization. *Journal of Advanced Nursing*. 2002; **39**(4): 325–32.
2. Culliford L. *The Psychology of Spirituality: an Introduction*. London: Jessica Kingsley, 2011.
3. Holy Bible. Job; 42:12. King James edition. London: Printed by Eyre and Spottiswoode Ltd; Pre 1929.
4. Nekolaichuk CL, Jevne RF and Maguire TO. Structuring the meaning of hope in health and illness. *Social Science and Medicine*. 1999; **48**: 591–605.
5. Flemming K. The meaning of hope to palliative care patients. *International Journal of Palliative Nursing*. 1997; **3**(1): 14–8.
6. Bingley AF, McDermott E, Thomas C *et al*. Making sense of dying: a review of narratives written since 1950 by people facing death from cancer and other diseases. *Palliative Medicine*. 2006; **20**(3): 183–95.
7. Sheldon F. *Psychosocial Palliative Care*. Cheltenham; Stanley Thornes, 1997.
8. Stanworth R. *Recognising Spiritual Needs in People Who Are Dying*. Oxford: Oxford University Press, 2004.
9. Adams H. Art as Therapy. In: Greenstreet W, editor. *Integrating Spirituality in Health and Social Care: Perspectives and Practical Approaches*. Oxford: Radcliffe Publishing, 2006, 139–50.
10. Holloway M. *Negotiating Death in Contemporary Health and Social Care*. Bristol: Policy Press, 2007.
11. Webb P. Advocacy. In: Webb P, editor. *Ethical Issues in Palliative Care: Reflections and Considerations*. Manchester: Hochland and Hochland, 2000, 65–80.
12. Jeffery D. Care versus cure. In: Webb P, editor. *Ethical Issues in Palliative Care: Reflections and Considerations*. Manchester: Hochland and Hochland, 2000, 15–42.
13. Randall F and Downie RS. *The Philosophy of Palliative Care: Critique and Reconstruction*. Oxford: Oxford University Press, 2006.
14. Ibid.

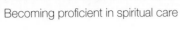
15. Thomas K. *Caring for the Dying at Home: Companions on the Journey.* Oxford: Radcliffe Medical Press, 2003.

16. Bury M. Illness narratives: fact or fiction? *Sociology of Health and Illness.* 2001; **23**(3): 263–85.

17. Ballhausen Footman E. The loss adjusters. *Mortality.* 1998; **3**(3): 291–5.

18. Sheldon, op. cit.

19. Golsworthy R and Coyle A. Spiritual beliefs and the search for meaning among older adults following partner loss. *Mortality.* 1999; **4**(1): 21- 40.

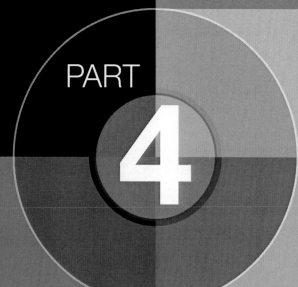

PART 4

IMPLICATIONS FOR EDUCATION AND PRACTICE

Every person is considered to have a spiritual dimension, albeit not necessarily one that they have developed or are able to recognize.[1] Spirituality is not an intellectual exercise but a lived experience,[2] and as such its development contributes to a person's awareness or consciousness of spiritual matters. Nurses who 'become' more spiritually mature are more likely to be able to help patients engage with spirituality as a resource.

There were four overriding ways in which participant experience illustrated how use and development of spiritual resources helped them cope with recurrent exposure to loss, as well as support patients' spiritual needs in end of life care.

- Fundamental to nurses' coping with the emotional demands of end of life care and their spiritual development was belonging to a work culture that permitted cultivation and nurture of spirituality and so enabled reciprocal peer support. Belief in hospice philosophy imbued end of life care practice with a sense of living 'in hope'.
- The relevance of belief in making sense of situations of loss was evident for both nurse and patient. Study findings imply that nurses not only needed to clarify their own spiritual stance if they are to support patients in spiritual care, but would benefit from a more in-depth understanding of the role of belief in meaning making. Improved understanding may enhance their spiritual development and provision of spiritual care.
- The nature of the nurse–patient relationship and the means of communication demonstrated a certain way of nurses 'being' with their patients that constituted spiritual caring. 'Openness' as a particular style of communication within nurse–patient relationships involved sharing of self and connecting with something deeper in patients. The implication from study findings is that this open style of communication can be learnt, and thus contribute to nurses' spiritual development and proficiency in care.

- Nurses who develop the means of protecting themselves, who address their own emotional needs and are therefore able to cope with the trauma of end of life care, reflect a maturity that enables them to become deeply involved in caring for patients in situations of loss. The implication for developing spiritual maturity is therefore discipline in self-care.

REFERENCES

1. Jewell A, editor. Introduction. *Spirituality and Personhood in Dementia*. London: Jessica Kingsley, 2011, 13–29.
2. Wright SG. Faith, hope, and clarity. *Nursing Standard*. 2002; **17**(6): 22–3.

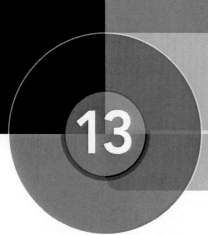

Work culture

13

If nurses are to offer spiritual care it is vital that they too receive appropriate care.[1] Study findings illustrate a paradox in the availability and need for support in different end of life care settings. However, each practice setting imbued hospice philosophy in its end of life practice. This philosophy provided nurses with a sense of living 'in hope' in situations of loss.

RESOLVING THE PARADOX: SUPPORT IN DIFFERENT END OF LIFE CARE SETTINGS

Hospice nurses' experience of end of life care is 'intensive' in that all patients are terminally ill and many have challenging symptoms. Fortunately, the ratio of registered nurses is high and so the potential for peer support availability at any one time is strong. Community nurse experience of end of life care is strengthening as health policy changes to accommodate sicker patients living longer.[2] As a consequence, increasing numbers of patients with complex needs are being cared for at home for longer, rather than being admitted for institutional care. The ratio of registered nurses to patients is therefore relatively robust, but the availability of peer support is more nebulous in that it is sourced by catching colleagues 'back at the office'. Nurses employed in the nursing home accommodate patients' gradual decline into end of life situations with staffing ratios primarily designed for general care. Registered nurses would bring some experience of situations of loss to the nursing home, given that pre-registration education of nurses inevitably involves encounters with situations where patients are dying or where death actually occurs. However, the presence of any experience is diluted by support workers who have not necessarily had any experience of end of life care. Consequently, when patients are in the advanced stage of a chronic illness the responsibility for support falls heavily on the registered nurse in charge of 'the floor' at the time. Any peer support the registered nurse might need due to the emotional demands of end of like care situations is delayed due to low ratio and the location of other registered nurses on different floors.

Therefore as the intensity of facing the challenges of end of life care is reduced across practice environments, so is the experience of staff in dealing with these situations, and yet it is in these settings that nurse peers as a source of support are mostly a virtual presence. Hence a significant implication for practice is the need to strengthen a collegial team ethos of support in community and nursing home settings. This can be achieved through effective use of clinical supervision.

Clinical supervision if performed well is comprehensive in the nature of support that it can generate.[3,4] The supervision given by a deputy manager was described by one research participant as not being of 'very good quality' and may reflect the supervisor's failure to fully understand or address the potential of this activity. Issues of measurable, outcome-driven practice exemplify what Schon[5] describes as problems of the 'high ground'. These are manageable as solutions lend themselves to research-based theory and technique. However, questions for exploration in those seeking restorative support are more likely to be from what Schon[6] describes as the 'swampy lowland', where messy, confusing problems of greatest human concern defy technical solution. Managerial agendas major in the technicalities of efficient and effective care. However, it is particularly important that the less technical, messy issues of restorative function addressing occupational stressors are dealt with in end of life care practice.

In contrast, the enthusiastic description of group supervision by another participant clearly indicated how very much this had been valued. The group was interprofessional and well attended. Its strength in being chaired by a clinical psychologist from outside the institution avoided any power issues that potentially inhibit group function[7] and thus cemented the collegiality of the group. Unfortunately, this also proved to be the group's weakness, in that the cost of buying in an outside chairperson became prohibitive and resulted in its demise.

This example illustrates how group supervision might provide the means of promoting and strengthening collegial support in the nursing home and community nursing teams. Key to authentic use of supervision as restorative support is the effective preparation of a practitioner committed to the ideals of the role, rather than it being left to line management as a token of compliance to an acknowledged need. Collegiality would be embedded if a member of the nursing team was suitably prepared. This would also not incur the prohibitive cost of buying in an outside facilitator.

Johns[8] outlines the characteristics and skills needed by a clinical supervisor to create a climate in which a practitioner can feel safe to disclose experiences they would like to explore. An important factor is the arrangements for supervision. The contract between participants is negotiated so that the frequency and expectations of supervision as well as the means of monitoring development are clear from the start. The responsibilities of those taking part are also established, the practitioner(s) determining the subject for guided reflection and the supervisor nurturing the practitioners' acceptance of this responsibility and consequently also accepting responsibility for monitoring their own practice.

The skills of supervision are not dissimilar to those needed in developing trust and rapport with patients (see Chapter 11). The supervisor's presence needs to be supportive and open to entering into and understanding the practitioner's perspective. This supportive ambience is necessary for practitioners to feel safe enough to disclose their thoughts in reflective dialogue. In establishing a rapport the supervisor is more likely to be able to interpret what the practitioner is meaning and respond appropriately. Active listening provides cues for the supervisor to guide exploratory conversation that endeavours to reveal details relevant to the subject/situation that the practitioner has brought to the session. A high level of support is required if the supervisor finds it necessary to confront the practitioner with the need to face and resolve contradiction on their part.

Johns[9] explains that there are a number of lenses or frames used to structure learning through reflection. These are a helpful guide for the supervisor. Initially, the practitioners' beliefs and values about nursing may need to be clarified, for example in relation to what they mean by terms they use, such as 'effective' practice. Similarly, practitioner understanding of the accountability and responsibility inherent in their role may be relevant to the situation being considered. Reflection on the knowledge that guided the practitioners in the situation, or on research or literature that might have helped, promotes absorption and integration of worth-while theory into patterns of knowing in practice. If the practitioner could not take the action they felt appropriate, they need to be encouraged to reflect on the reasons for this in relation to the reality of the limitations within their work culture and thus avoid unrealistic expectation of themselves. The situation may be considered in relation to similar past experiences in order to help problem identification and resolution through that experience.

LIVING 'IN HOPE' IN SITUATIONS OF LOSS

In a study by Dufault and Martocchio[10] hope is described as constituting two different spheres: generalized hope, which provides a sense of something beneficial to come, and particularized hope, focused on a particular goal in expectation of improvement. Data collected by participant observation over a period of two years of 35 elderly people (over 65 years of age) with cancer was analysed. Results were confirmed by analysis of further data from 47 terminally ill patients (14 years and older) with varied diagnoses, again collected over a two-year period. Although this study was carried out some time ago, and is not generalizable due to the nature and size of samples, its value is acknowledged in more recent research.[11] Generalized hope was found to protect against despair in situations that deprived people of particular hopes[12] and therefore is very relevant to end of life care contexts. It is rather nebulous in that it provides a positive glow (rather than a particular hope) that drives motivation to carry on, to persevere. Hence, general-ized hope provides a way of living 'in hope'.

Participants' sense of living 'in hope' seemed to be driven by the integration of hospice phi-losophy in their end of life care practice. All but one participant had undertaken post-registration study to enhance their understanding of hospice philosophy. Focused on improving quality of care and holistic in nature, hospice philosophy incorporates the physical, psychological, social and spiritual needs of individual patients.[13] The positive focus of care on the facilitation of 'living' until the event of death can generate generalized hope. This is exemplified in Barnard et al.'s[14] phenomenological study of palliative nursing, in which participants described how encounters with life-limiting illness increased their appreciation of valuing each day. Similarly, in research by Webster and Kristjanson,[15] descriptions given by staff with long-term experience of caring for the terminally ill implied a sense of vitality, a way of living.

Hospice philosophy incorporates not only the concept of holistic care in practice, but also a commitment to the dissemination and development of end of life care practice through educa-tion and research.[16] One of the values of education in hospice philosophy is the development of a belief in a different style of practice. This comprises a shift in world view that embraces the paradox of end of life care in acknowledging that the extremely harrowing can be very reward-ing.[17] In this way, a professional world view primarily focused on the recovery of patients, which generates an attitude of 'there's nothing more than we can do' in situations of end of life care, shifts to one of living in hope of 'there is always something that can be done'. Ultimately, this may be the therapeutic sharing of self as one human being with another. In this way, nurses use their hope of helping as a spiritual resource. Participants benefited from accessing local hospice educational provision, which taught the fundaments of this philosophy. Some nurses went on to more comprehensive study to achieve higher education awards in, or relevant to, end of life care practice. Consequently, the continued provision of unaccredited courses by local hospices is an invaluable resource in either initiating or affirming an understanding of hospice philoso-phy and holistic practice, as well as potentially generating motivation for further development in end of life care practice.

SUMMARY

Collegial relationships within nursing teams are described as similar to a family in that they involve people with different personality types, different ages, different backgrounds and different experiences who care and support each other.[18] In belonging to supportive teams nurses are able to share and explore the meaning of their experiences with their colleagues. Where face-to-face exploration is limited due to logistics, teamworking patterns and skill mix, collegial support can potentially be enhanced by group supervision facilitated by a suitably prepared practitioner.

Barnard *et al.*[19] suggest that finding meaning in caring for people with terminal and advanced chronic illness involves searching for meaning in nursing practice and the experience of others. The value of education in the fundaments of holistic philosophy are evident in promoting a work culture that embraces a positive focus of care on the facilitation of 'living' until the event of death. This generates an attitude of living in hope that 'there is always something that can be done' and is one that enables nurses to find meaning in their nursing practice, to use their hope of helping as a spiritual resource.

REFERENCES

1. Morrison P and Burnard P. *Caring and Communicating: the Interpersonal Relationship in Nursing.* Chichester: Macmillan, 1991.
2. Thomas K. *Caring for the Dying at Home: Companions on the Journey.* Oxford: Radcliffe Medical Press, 2003.
3. Nicklin P. A practice-centred model of clinical supervision. *Nursing Times.* 1997. **93**(46): 52–4.
4. Johns C. *Becoming a Reflective Practitioner.* Oxford: Blackwell Science, 2000.
5. Schon DA. *Educating the Reflective Practitioner.* San Francisco, CA: Jossey-Bass, 1987.
6. Ibid.
7. Hall P. Interprofessional teamwork: professional cultures as barriers. *Journal of Interprofessional Care.* 2005; Supplement **1**: 188–96.
8. Johns, op. cit.
9. Ibid.
10. Dufault K and Martocchio B. Hope: its spheres and dimensions. *Nursing Clinics of North American.* 1985; **20**: 379–91.
11. Nekolaichuk CL, Jevne RF and Maguire TO. Structuring the meaning of hope in health and illness. *Social Science and Medicine.* 1999; **48**: 591–605.
12. Dufault and Martocchio, op. cit.
13. Sepulveda C, Marlin A, Yoshida T *et al.* Palliative care: the World Health Organisation's global perspective. *Journal of Pain and Symptom Management.* 2002; **24**(2): 91–6.
14. Barnard A, Hollingum C and Hartfiel B. Going on a journey: understanding palliative nursing. *International Journal of Palliative Nursing.* 2006; **12**(1): 6–12.
15. Webster J and Kristjanson LJ. 'But isn't it depressing?': the vitality of palliative care. *Journal of Palliative Care.* 2002; **18**(1): 15–24.
16. Twycross R. *Introducing Palliative Care.* Oxford: Radcliffe Medical Press, 1999.
17. Ibid.
18. Barnard, Hollingum and Hartfiel, op. cit.
19. Ibid.

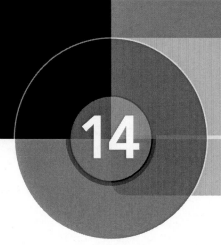

Role of belief in meaning making

14

Educational settings provide the space for initiating either reflection on, or review of, personal spiritual stance. Study findings demonstrate that belief has been a significant resource in research participants' experience of loss, and has impacted their aptitude for care. Consequently, rather than just being encouraged to clarify their own spiritual stance, nurses may also benefit from a more extensive exploration of the role of belief in meaning making. If, for example, participants had shared their narratives of spiritual journey in an educational forum they would have known that their stories followed a similar pattern. Understanding patterns of belief may develop their ability to recognize this in others. Review of literature and research that illuminates the complexity of the human need to search for meaning, as well as tools such as narrative that facilitate meaning making, would enhance nurses' theoretical base for spiritual development of practice. This chapter considers material that might facilitate such development.

THE LINK BETWEEN BELIEF AND MEANING

In their hermeneutic study that explored the meaning of spirituality and spiritual care, McLeod and Wright[1] define belief in terms of what is taken to be true. In 12 therapeutic conversations with three families living with serious illness, they found that belief could facilitate health and healing if it helped family members find some meaning that they could live with, whereas meaninglessness created suffering. McLeod and Wright's[2] study therefore illustrates the role of belief in meaning making.

THE SEARCH FOR MEANING

Establishing belief is a complex process impacted by individual development and experience. The search to understand either meaning of immediate circumstances or the meaning of life itself can be triggered in situations of significant loss.

The narratives of the spiritual journey given by several participants described how they have arrived at their current belief. Involved in religious communities in their childhood, religious belief had been external and needed to be 'learnt' by each child. Some spoke of their rejection of religion and others sought their own interpretation of religious faith as they moved toward adolescence and early adulthood. This shared similarity of pattern of development of belief that involved challenging what they had been taught to believe was not evident to participants themselves, nor was it recognized in patient assessment. There are a number of different perspectives on why the pattern of development of belief follows a similar pattern:

MAN'S SEARCH FOR MEANING

Frankl[3] believes that man's search for meaning is the primary motivation in life. Hence the rejection of religion may reflect the intrinsic need for individual participants to search and discover for themselves how they are to make sense of existential questions, even if ultimately they find their answers in the organized beliefs of the religious community they rejected. Participants' search contributed to the clarity of their personal spiritual stance. This clarity promotes nurses' spiritual integrity when caring for vulnerable and distressed patients.[4]

THE IMPACT OF EDUCATION ON SPIRITUALITY AS MEANING AND 'RELATIONAL CONSCIOUSNESS'

The timing of a decline in religious or spiritual interest appears to coincide with children's introduction to the traditions of science, often accompanied by religious skepticism.[5] The impact of contradictory educational influences is supported, at least in part, by Hay and Nye's[6] grounded theory study of children's spirituality.

Their study involved 38 children who attended primary school in two industrial cities in the English Midlands. Children were randomly selected (subject to the proviso that samples included an equal number of boys and girls); 18 were 6–7 years old and 20 were 10–11 years old. Approximately three quarters of the children were classified as having no religious affiliation. Hay discusses at length the challenge of talking to children about spirituality. The outcome was that Nye spent time in the primary schools so that she became a familiar figure to the children. She also invited each child to tell her about their life and interests at the beginning of meetings, in order to put the children at their ease, before moving on to a focus on spirituality. This shift in conversation was triggered by the use of photographs chosen to generate awareness, value or mystery sensing, for example a photograph of a child gazing into a fire, or of a child starring at a dead pet. After listening to the child's reflections on these images Nye encouraged the children to share any similar experiences of their own.

Up to three meetings of about half an hour were conducted with each of the children. Following the analysis of tapes that recorded these conversations, Nye describes the core of children's spirituality as relational consciousness. Excerpts of conversations illustrated that spirituality was experienced through a child's 'sense of' relationship with the natural world, to others, to God, with their own identity and their own mental life. Hay goes on to suggest that spirituality expressed as relational consciousness is an ever-present aspect of being human, a holistic 'sense' or 'direct knowledge of', separate from and prior to intellectual 'knowledge about' phenomena. Hay considers the primal nature of relational consciousness accounts for why it can be seen particularly clearly in children. In pre-dating intellectual analysis it constitutes an awareness of our link with what is described as the seamless robe of reality, our implicit awareness that damage to any part of reality is damage to the fabric of which we are a part. In this way, self-sacrificing behaviour for others is seen as a function of spiritual awareness. This concept is not dissimilar to nurses partaking in the sharing of self in professional contexts, described by Campbell[7] as 'moderated love' and by Bradshaw[8] as covenantal care, and so the participants who described experiences that reflect this style of practice appear to have sustained something of their relational consciousness. However, Hay's concern, regardless of whether individual convictions are religious or secular, is that our society's culture of individualism promotes self-interest, which undermines human relational consciousness and so 'blots out' the holistic nature of spiritual awareness. Similarly, contractual care may 'blot out' spiritual awareness, in much the same way as participants described colleagues who were focused on task efficiency rather than establishing patient rapport.

CONSTRUCTING MEANINGS AND GROWTH OF THE SELF

Critical distancing and re-approaching religion is attributed by Kezdy et al.[9] to a change in attitude to religiosity. In their review of literature in preparation for a cross-sectional survey investigating religious doubt and mental health they described different approaches to religion. First, there is the choice of acceptance or rejection of a belief in a transcendent reality. For those who accept the existence of a God, the way in which religion is approached can be either literal or symbolic. A literal approach reflects a preference for clarity rather than ambiguity, and assumes that there is only one right answer for each problem. A symbolic approach, on the other hand, is determined by different cognitive variables, such as open-mindedness and tolerance of ambiguity. Kezdy et al.[10] suggest these approaches to religion are reflected in Fowler's[11] theoretical model of faith, which draws on cognitive,[12] moral[13] and personality[14] staged models of development. He describes the development of faith across the lifespan as having six stages, with few people reaching the final stage.[15] Fowler's second stage of faith development is one that spans school years in which beliefs are expressed as literal interpretations. The stimulus to move on to the third stage, associated with adolescence, is the occurrence of contradictions in these literal interpretations that require reflection on meanings. Such reflection demonstrates the changes in the complexity of thinking in adolescence that are necessary for symbolic interpretation. Fowler's further stages of faith development reflect an increasing relevance of an ability to tolerate uncertainties and accommodate paradox as an aspect of faith in adulthood. This growth is ongoing and evident in the different stages of spiritual maturity reflected in participant stories. Spiritual maturity in nurses promotes proficiency in spiritual care.

NARRATIVE AS A TOOL FOR MEANING MAKING

The recognition by one nurse of repetition of illness narratives by patients as a route to healing, and the insights that became apparent to several nurses when relating the story of their own experience, are all examples of ways in which narrative works in relation to meaning making.

This process of meaning making is described by Carrithers[16] as narrative thought. He explains that narrative thought simultaneously involves action, for example the situation I find myself in, and consciousness, such as the way I feel and what I know or do not know about that. It involves not only our knowledge and awareness of our immediate relation with another person, but also the many human interactions we have had over a period of considerable time. In this way it allows us to understand complex action and to act appropriately. Hence, narrative thought is more than a means of telling stories, as it also provides a way of understanding involved, intricate situations and attitudes. Narrative therefore provides a potential tool for nurses and patients, a spiritual resource, in that it facilitates making sense of situations.

MEANING MADE OVER TIME, 'RETROSPECTIVE REAPPRAISAL' AND FORGIVENESS

O'Connor[17] reviewed available research, theoretical and empirical evidence on adjustment to negative life events. She explains that in order to find meaning in an event we explore the significance of the event in our lives overall. Meaning can be made over time by 'retrospective reappraisal'.[18] Social sharing of feelings and reactions in conversation with supportive others has been found to positively benefit those impacted by the emotional disruptiveness of an event.[19]

O'Connor[20] goes on to propose a meaning-making model that could explain adjustment to loss. Meaning making is considered as a marriage of emotion and cognition, with meaning described as an important crossroads that allows us to move from negative emotion, due for example to loss, through a cognitive understanding of the event, to positive emotion. In this way, the event does not merely have negative repercussions but positive ones as well, such as the positive sense of achievement by nurses in getting what dying patients want right, despite the loss of the patient through death.

This shift from a negative to positive emotion through cognitive reappraisal of the situation is similar to the concept of forgiveness, in which a past event, which cannot be altered, can be seen in a fresh light.[21,22,23] The capacity to forgive oneself, to live with one's flaws,[24] is as important a spiritual need as forgiving another. Formally promoting an understanding of the concepts of forgiveness and retrospective reappraisal would contribute to proficiency in spiritual care in that they would raise nurses' awareness, and thus potential sensitivity, to issues of guilt as a source of spiritual distress. Several research participants demonstrated this proficiency in describing situations where they were able to sense issues of distress related to patients' estranged relationships or personal history. Such understanding is invaluable in that it promotes optimism in offering possible ways of helping patients in distress.

CONGRUENCE AS A CONCEPT FACILITATING MEANING

Western culture predominantly values control, and as science and technology have moved the capabilities of medicine forward, this has driven an expectation of people living to adulthood, and beyond to an increasingly old age. It is therefore not surprising that participants found it difficult to deal with young, untimely deaths. Friedemann *et al.*[25] advocate a more congruent philosophy of health in which human control is balanced with spirituality as an alternative means of coping. Certainly some nurses used personal philosophy or faith to process and make sense of situations of loss. This ability to transcend difficult circumstances exemplifies the development of spiritual maturity.

SUMMARY

Our search for meaning as a primary motivation in life is honed in situations of loss. Sources of individual belief can facilitate meaning making and so contribute to both healing for patients and a clarity for nurses that strengthens their spiritual integrity. Education that explores different perspectives and patterns of the development of belief can benefit nurses in their understanding of the relationship between belief and meaning, and therefore enhance their theoretical base for the spiritual development of practice. The concepts of 'moderated love' and covenantal care provide material that exemplifies human intuitive relational consciousness as holistic spiritual awareness. Spiritual maturity, both in nurses and in their patients, may be considered in terms of stages of faith that reflect the dynamics of how they have made sense of difficult situations they have faced over time. Helping nurses to understand how narrative provides a tool for meaning making engenders a further spiritual resource for care. Education that encourages an understanding of the concepts of forgiveness and retrospective reappraisal empowers nurses to promote optimism in offering potential ways of helping patients in distress, and in this way to develop proficiency in spiritual care.

REFERENCES

1. McLeod DL and Wright LM. Living the as-yet unanswered: spiritual care practices in family systems nursing. *Journal of Family Nursing*. 2008; **14**(1): 118–41.
2. Ibid.
3. Frankl VE. *Man's Search for Meaning*. New York: Washington Square Press, 1984.
4. Cornette K. For whenever I am weak, I am strong… *International Journal of Palliative Nursing*. 1997; **3**(1): 6–13.
5. Culliford L. *The Psychology of Spirituality: an Introduction*. London: Jessica Kingsley, 2011.
6. Hay D, Nye R. *The Spirit of the Child*. London: Jessica Kingsley, 2006.
7. Campbell A. *Moderated Love: a Theology of Professional Care*. London: SPCK, 1984.
8. Bradshaw A. *Lighting the Lamp: the Spiritual Dimension of Nursing Care*. Harrow: Scutari Press, 1994.
9. Kezdy A, Martos T, Boland V *et al*. Religious doubts and mental health in adolescence and young adulthood: the association with religious attitudes. *Journal of Adolescence*. 2011; **34**: 39–47.
10. Ibid.
11. Fowler JW. *Stages of Faith: the Psychology of Human Development and the Quest for Meaning*. Philadelphia: Harper Row, 1981.
12. Piaget J. *Six Psychological Studies*. New York: Random House, 1967.
13. Kohlberg L. Education, moral development, and faith. *Journal of Moral Education*. 1974; **4**(1): 5–16.
14. Erikson EH. *Childhood and Society*. New York: Norton, 1963.
15. Greenstreet W. Clarifying the concept. In: Greenstreet W, editor. *Integrating Spirituality in Health and Social Care: Perspectives and Practical Approaches*. Oxford: Radcliffe Publishing, 2006, 7–19.
16. Carrithers M. *Why Humans Have Cultures: Explaining Anthropology and Social Diversity*. Oxford: Oxford University Press, 1992.
17. O'Connor M-F. Making meaning of life events: theory, evidence, and research directions for an alternative model. *Omega*. 2002; **46**(1): 51–75.
18. Bonanno GA, Kaltman S. Toward an integrative perspective on bereavement. *Psychological Bulletin*. 1999; **125**: 760–76.
19. Rime B, Mesquita B, Philippot P *et al*. Beyond the emotional event: six studies on the social sharing of emotion. *Cognition and Emotion*. 1991; **5**: 435–65.
20. O'Connor, op. cit.

21. Saunders C. *Living with Dying: a Guide to Palliative Care*. Oxford: Oxford University Press, 1995.

22. Stanworth R. Attention: a potential vehicle for spiritual care. *Journal of Palliative Care*. 2002; **18**(3): 192–5.

23. McCullough ME, Root LM, Cohen AD. Writing about the benefits of an interpersonal transgression facilitates forgiveness. *Journal of Consulting and Clinical Psychology*. 2006; **74**(5): 887–97.

24. Myco F. The non-believer in the health care situation. In: McGilloway O, Myco F, editors. *Nursing and Spiritual Care*. London: Harper and Row, 1985, 36–52.

25. Friedemann M, Mouch J and Racey T. Nursing the spirit: the framework of systemic organization. *Journal of Advanced Nursing*. 2002; **39**(4): 325–32.

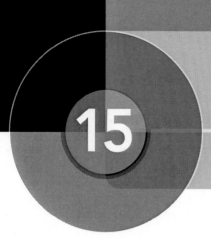

'Openness' as a particular style of communication

15

Being available as a spiritual resource is rooted in what Morse *et al.*[1] describe as reflexive or 'connected' response to human suffering, such as consolation, compassion and commiseration. These automatic responses are culturally conditioned and exist prior to formal preparation to nurse. Therefore a strong emphasis on the value of maintaining or recapturing this predisposition to reflexive response needs to be included in teaching and developing communication skills in professional practice.

ISSUES OF STYLE IN COMMUNICATION

Spiritual care in end of life contexts necessitates nurses 'staying with' those who are suffering, and so risks involvement. Morse *et al.*[2] used autobiographical and biographical accounts of caregiver and patient interaction to illustrate their model of communication, which describes nurses' responses to patients who are suffering. They differentiate between nurses' communication as a connected response and alternative distancing strategies.

CONNECTED COMMUNICATION

Empathetic insight by the nurse, triggered by suffering, can open therapeutic use of communication that involves active listening. Patients reciprocate in becoming more open in what they share as they warm to the sense of being valued. Morse *et al.*[3] suggest that empathetic insight into suffering pre-dates professional learning and in this way therapeutic communication as a connected response may be linked to relational consciousness (see Chapter 14). Participant accounts provide numerous examples of engagement with suffering through 'connected' responses, together with evidence that sharing of self in this way is emotionally demanding.

'EFFICIENCY' AND 'CHATTER'; ESCAPING REAL LIFE AND DEATH ISSUES

Nurses or carers who resort to false reassurance to distance themselves from suffering or use a form of pseudo-engagement, a learned professional response as a means of protecting themselves, are unlikely to be open to patient cues indicating they have something difficult to ask or share, but instead close down any opportunities they have of understanding patients' deep-seated needs. Research participant responses described some nurses as focused on efficiency and task. This approach is one of contractual care that fails to attempt a connected response. Shortfalls in style of communication were considered remedial through education. However, if the root of connected communication is seated in empathetic insight into suffering that pre-dates professional learning, educational settings will need to be experiential, in order to open up the possibility of rediscovery. Culliford,[4] for example, describes the experiential activities of medical students learning to take a spiritual history as a means of improving listening and offering what he calls 'deep presence'. The process was one of conversation while 'watching' people for visual clues, as well as well as setting the emotional tone of information. Students found a gentle, unhurried approach best. This style of approach is also thought to have a beneficial therapeutic effect, a possible reciprocal empathy where the patient senses warmth and positivity in medical staff, in much the same way as described above. Culliford[5] advocates the potential benefit of all health and social care professionals engaging with patients in this way.

A potential coping strategy used in situations of loss is the use of everyday 'chatter' to escape the real life and death issues that these circumstances tend to throw up. Support workers were seen to use 'chatter' to distract themselves or the patient from an issue that is a matter of concern. They were also described as tending to consider their role as one of tasks to complete rather having a more vocational view of caring. The need for support workers to grow and 'become' more spiritually aware in their delivery of care was addressed by establishing a reflection group, in which they were encouraged to share experiences. The group not only provided the opportunity to consider the development of more therapeutic communication skills, but also provided an opportunity to tease out existential issues that present themselves when caring for the dying. This reflection group evidences a clinically based means of 'how' to raise spiritual awareness and promote competence in spiritual care.

MEANS OF COMMUNICATION

Heidegger's[6] idea of 'Being' is one that reflects the 'essence' of our human existence (see Chapter 2). Communication is a key element of our 'Being' and in our spiritual care of others. Heidegger[7] further describes 'Being' as the quiet power of the possible, in that it presides over thinking. In thinking 'Being' comes to language and therefore is both manifested and maintained in language through speech. However, the flexibility and the multidimensionality peculiar to thinking is difficult to maintain as language complies with expedient communication within a public realm, where what is considered intelligible and unintelligible is already decided. Only in alternative forms of communication such as poetic creation or metaphor can spoken language mimic thinking in being liberated from grammar.

Metaphor conveys a 'sense of' rather than direct meaning. It does this by comparing the unfamiliar with the familiar, but also seeks to establish familiarity between speaker and listener. In expressing what is difficult to put into words, the speaker uses metaphor as an invitation for the hearer to make a special effort to accept, and so share, 'a sense of' what the speaker is trying to convey.[8] On occasion some participants used metaphor to convey meaning. In doing so, they reflected their potential to understand metaphor, to listen for multidimensional thought and associated sensitivity, to the essence of meaning being conveyed when patients find conventional grammar falls short in the expression of spiritual matters. Nurses' understanding of the use of metaphor and sensitivity to others' use of metaphor is a valuable asset in spiritual care and worthy of some exploration in educational forums.

SUMMARY

'Openness' as a particular style of communication is facilitated by experiential learning. The skills that enable therapeutic nursing presence are developed in much the same way as Culliford[9] describes the experiential activities of medical students. Deep presence is achieved through active listening, watching for visual clues and setting the emotional tone of conversation with patients. Clinically based reflection groups to raise spiritual awareness are another means of promoting competence in spiritual care. An exploration and understanding of the use of metaphor where language falls short in expressing spiritual and existential concerns may be of value.

REFERENCES

1. Morse JM, Bottorff J, Anderson G *et al.* Beyond empathy: expanding expressions of caring. *Journal of Advanced Nursing.* 1992; **17**: 809–21.
2. Ibid.
3. Ibid.
4. Culliford L. *The Psychology of Spirituality: an Introduction.* London: Jessica Kingsley, 2011.
5. Ibid.
6. Heidegger M. 1967 Letter on Humanism. In: Farrell Krell D, editor. *Martin Heidegger Basic Writings.* London: Routledge, 1993, 217–65.
7. Ibid.
8. Madsen C. *The Bones Reassembled: Reconstituting Liturgical Speech.* Aurora: Davies Group, 2005.
9. Culliford, op. cit.

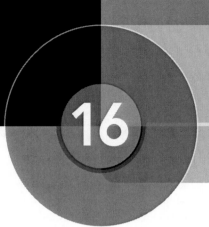

Discipline in self-care

The learned ability to cope with psychic and physical challenges in situations of caring is described by Finfgeld-Connett[1] as professional maturity. Professionally mature spiritual care involves nurses developing the ability to protect themselves, to maintain a healthy emotional balance and so manage their involvement in therapeutic relationships with patients. It requires balancing professional practice and personal life, acknowledging personal vulnerability and owning the need for support as well as being disciplined in taking time out for spiritual replenishment. Professional growth that culminates in such maturity comes with experience in nursing practice as well as life experience. However, educational settings provide a forum for raising an awareness of the importance of balancing professional practice and personal life, as well as a safe haven for the means of achieving this to be shared or discussed.

PROFESSIONAL GROWTH IN EXPERIENCE

One nurse was explicit, and others implied, that the ability to persevere in the face of recurrent situations of loss was due to the development of life skills, sourced from the experience of encounter rather than taught. This view is supported in published literature. Dirkx et al.,[2] for example, explain that transformative, deep learning challenges existing assumptions and integrates our experiences of the outer world with the experience of our inner worlds. In this way, significantly novel dilemmas effect learning through critical reflection by changing meaning and perspective.[3] Critical reflection benefits from a structured approach.[4] Education can contribute to professional growth by empowering nurses with the skills to choose and use a model of reflection that best suits their mindset.

Nursing requires a particular mode of knowing, one that is sensitive to situations and the appropriate response.[5] This mode of knowing or 'tact' is tacit in that it is not drawn from principles but from practical knowledge.[6] It accounts for participants' ability to sense a patient's need without understanding why. Professionals experienced at being open in the presence of a patient learn to feel their feelings, to trust intuitive thinking that takes place below awareness, a form of non-discursive thought that occurs as the conscious mind processes the experience.[7] Therefore, 'openness' as a particular style of communication (see Chapter 15) facilitates growth in nurses' 'tacit knowing'.

PERSONAL GROWTH IN BEREAVEMENT

Stories of life-changing personal loss and negative experience were found to contribute to a positive development of self, and a better understanding of patient and family situations in practice. These experiences reflect a growth in resilience following biographical disruption,[8] as time effects a shift from emotional upheaval to coping.

Folkman's[9] study of care-giving partners found the common theme associated with positive psychological states for those coping with severe stress was searching for and finding positive meaning in the event. Meaning is created by finding a redeeming value in significant loss. Nurses who had suffered a personal bereavement discovered a new clarity, a new depth of understanding of grief. Lloyd[10] supports these nurses' claim to be in a better place in empathising with patients and relatives in end of life care contexts, because resilient professionals are more likely to promote resilience in others by being present and able to use active listening skills in even the most difficult patient situations.

OWNING THE NEED FOR SUPPORT

Situations of patient loss rendered some nurses more aware of their own vulnerability as persons. When we are in the presence of another, the call to respond to the other is what Levinas[11] terms 'the Face'. Beneath all expressions adopted by 'the Face' is vulnerability, a steadfast exposure to invisible death in that mortality lies in the 'Other'. In looking into 'the Face' we grow, become more aware of humanity and know ourselves to be mutually vulnerable. This vulnerability was evident in participant descriptions of practice experience that included a raised awareness of their own mortality. It also triggered a comparison of the patient's family's situation and their own, or imagining themselves in the patient's situation. Recognition of vulnerability potentially challenges a person's ability to stay in situations of loss.[12] Owning the need for support, rather than expecting 'stoically' to keep such fear to oneself, is the better[13] and spiritually mature response to maintaining professional and personal integrity in situations of emotional duress. Such maturity was inferred in the variety of ways participants accessed support, particularly within their nursing team, and made explicit in relation to support for support workers who were less familiar with death, and so potentially more vulnerable.

SPIRITUAL REPLENISHMENT

Sheldon[14] explains that there are limits to working in end of life care contexts, boundaries that need to be adhered to if the professional is to preserve their own integrity and not get lost in another's spiritual distress. Maintaining a balance between their work and home life was one way in which participants maintained boundaries. Spiritual maturity was evident in participant responses that reflected their ability to 'spend time' in getting back to 'being themselves' outside of the work environment. These included activities that replenished self, such as pottering in the greenhouse or listening to music, as well as solitary activities to reconnect with self, such as walking the dog or, more formally, spending time in a retreat.

Humour was also a means participants used to maintain perspective and so preserve integrity in end of life care practice. Culliford[15] describes spiritual practice as any regular activity that promotes spiritual development. He suggests a range of spiritual skills that can be learnt (see

Table 16.1 Spiritual practices

Mainly religious	Belonging to a faith tradition
	Ritual practices/worship
	Meditation and prayer
	Reading scripture
	Listening to/playing/singing sacred music
	Pilgrimages and retreats
Mainly non-religious/ secular	Contemplation
	Yoga/tai chi/similar disciplined practices
	Maintaining physical health
	Contemplative reading of literature, poetry, philosophy etc
	Engaging with/enjoying nature
	Appreciation of the arts
	Engaging in creative activities/artistic pursuits
	Joining clubs and societies
	Co-operative group/team activities involving a special quality of fellowship
	Maintaining stable family relationships and friendships
	Acts of compassion

© Larry Culliford 2011. *The Psychology of Spirituality*. Reproduced by permission of Jessica Kingsley Publishers.

Table 16.1) and includes humour in his repertoire as a means of connecting with joy. He cites research that supports the physical, psychological and social benefits of humour, and explains that good humour is not all about laughter but radiates from the spiritually mature.

The importance of taking time out to reconnect with the self as a means of spiritual replenishment is easily stated, but not so easily achieved. What has to be 'done' in both work and home environments can consume time, leaving no space to 'be'. Education settings provide an opportunity to encourage discussion, which highlights the importance of a disciplined approach to spending time in activities that are spiritually replenishing, raises awareness of the many ways this may be achieved and emphasizes the value of such activity as a spiritual resource for personal growth and professional practice.

SUMMARY

Professional maturity reflects an ability by nurses to become deeply involved in caring for patients without succumbing to overemotional forms of helping.[16] It also involves nurses developing the means of protecting themselves, and maintaining a healthy ability to replenish and/or reconnect with self.

In various ways, and at different levels, participants exhibited professional maturity in their ability to 'get to know' their patients, and 'to stay' in working environments that were repeatedly emotionally challenging due to patients' loss and loss of patients. Contributory factors that enabled them to do this included an ability to recognize their own vulnerability and seek support, engaging in activities chosen for replenishment and solitary activity or 'time out' to just be themselves. In this way, they safeguarded their spiritual integrity, a crucial element in the development of proficiency in spiritual care.

REFERENCES

1. Finfgeld-Connett D. Meta-synthesis of caring in nursing. *Journal of Clinical Nursing*. 2008; **17**(2): 196–204.
2. Dirkx JM, Mezirow J and Cranton P. Musings and reflections on the meaning, context and process of transformative learning: a dialogue between John M. Dirkx and Jack Mezirow. *Journal of Transformative Education*. 2006; **4**(2): 123–39.
3. Mezirow J. Transformative learning: theory to practice. *New Directions for Adult Continuing Education*. 1997; **74**: 5–12.
4. Johns C. *Becoming a Reflective Practitioner*. Oxford: Blackwell Science, 2000.
5. McLeod DL and Wright LM. Living the as-yet unanswered: spiritual care practices in family systems nursing. *Journal of Family Nursing*. 2008; **14**(1): 118–41.
6. Benner P. The tradition and skill of interpretative phenomenology in studying health, illness, and caring practices. In: Benner P, editor. *Interpretive Phenomenology: Embodiment, Caring, and Ethics in Health and Illness*. Thousand Oaks, CA: Sage, 1994, 99–127.
7. Cassell E. Diagnosing suffering: a perspective. *Annals of Internal Medicine*. 1999; **131**(7): 531–4.
8. Bury M. Illness narratives: fact or fiction? *Sociology of Health and Illness*. 2001; **23**(3): 263–85.
9. Folkman S. Positive psychological states and coping with severe illness. *Social Science and Medicine*. 1997; **45**(8): 1207–21.
10. Lloyd M. Resilience promotion and its relevance to the personhood needs of people with dementia and other brain damage. In: Jewell A, editor. *Spirituality and Personhood in Dementia*. London: Jessica Kingsley, 2011, 141–52.
11. Levinas E. Ethics as first philosophy I–III. In: Hand S, editor. *The Levinas Reader*. Oxford: Blackwell, 1989, 75–82.
12. Sheldon F. *Psychosocial Palliative Care*. Cheltenham: Stanley Thornes, 1997.
13. Vachon M. Battle fatigue in hospice/palliative care. In: Gilmore A and Gilmore S, editors. *A Safer Death: Multidisciplinary Aspects of Terminal Care*. New York: Plenum, 1988.
14. Sheldon, op. cit.
15. Culliford L. *The Psychology of Spirituality: an Introduction*. London: Jessica Kingsley, 2011.
16. Euswas P. The actualized caring moment: a grounded theory of caring in nursing practice. In: Gaut DA, editor. *A Global Agenda for Caring*. New York: National League for Nursing, 1993, 309–26.

Index